#10 IN THE SERIES OF OUR
BOOKS YOU'LL ACTUALLY READ

FINDING
KETO

ANDREW EDWIN JENKINS

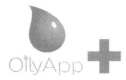
OilyApp +

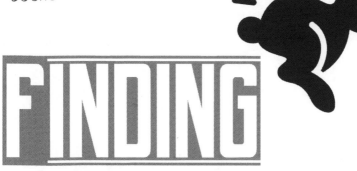

LOSE WEIGHT FAST
WITHOUT GOING HUNGRY.
WITHOUT GROWING TIRED. &
WITHOUT GETTING IRRITABLE

ISBN-13: 9781688461994

Connect online!

For general information go to the following websites >>>

Podcast- www. Jenkins.tv

Social-
www.Facebook.com/OilyApp
www.Instagram.com/OilyApp

Website-
www.OilyApp.com

Book webpage
FindingKeto.online

CONTENTS

PART 1 | KETO BASICS

PART 2 | YOUR PLAN & PRACTICAL TIPS

Access the audiobook + bonus content at www.FindingKeto.online

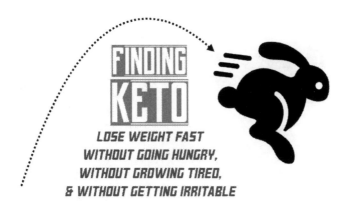

Access the audiobook + bonus content at www.FindingKeto.online

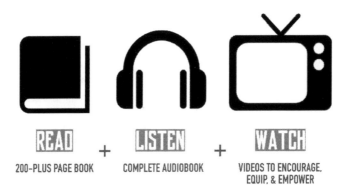

READ + **LISTEN** + **WATCH**

200-PLUS PAGE BOOK · COMPLETE AUDIOBOOK · VIDEOS TO ENCOURAGE, EQUIP, & EMPOWER

INTRO – BEEN THERE & DONE THAT

MAIN IDEA: I DID IT- YOU CAN, TOO.

Just a few years ago I was stressed out, overweight, pulling 80-hour work weeks, and aging way too fast. The emotional load of leading a church, a nonprofit, and being a husband and father kept me moving too fast. The days seemed long, yet the weeks seemed short. Incredibly short.

I remember looking across the bed more than once and asking my wife, as I fell asleep for the night, "Is it really *already* Thursday? Another week almost gone… *really*?"

Most of those conversations were smattered with questions about finances. We were living paycheck to paycheck. *Barely.* Most weeks consisted of transferring money right back out of savings that we'd just put in. Even at that, we had to decide if it was more important to pay the power bill or put gas in the car that week. Don't get me wrong: everything was always paid. But it didn't seem like we were living the "abundant life" you read about in the Bible. I was tired, I was unhealthy, and we were just scraping by.

During this season, I remembered the words the Apostle John prayed for the church when he was older. He blessed the church, saying, "I pray that you may prosper in all things and be in health, just as your soul prospers" (3 John 2 NKJV).

Right there, he assumed Jesus' followers were...

- Prospering in "all things" (maybe the topic of *another* book, OK?)

- Experiencing physical health (we'll discuss this throughout *this* book)

- Enjoying vitality of the soul (I talk about this on my podcast)[1]

At that time, I wasn't really experiencing *any* of the three things John prayed about!

Just how bad it was...

About five years ago my wife began building a business in the health and wellness industry, working from home. I didn't pay much attention to what she was doing until she won an all-expenses paid trip for two to Hawaii. Then, she had my attention!

We stayed in an incredible hotel while on the trip. And, relevant to this conversation, the resort's decor included a full length mirror in the bathroom- something we didn't have at home.

---

[1] Go to Jenkins.tv or search "The Overflow Podcast" on iTunes.

If you want to see how comfortable you really are in your own skin, go take a long stare at your self naked in a full length mirror. *I dare you.*

Anyway, I finished showering one night as we prepared to head to a dinner party. As I stepped out of the shower, I noticed myself in an over-sized bathroom mirror that hung over the double vanity (read: a mirror that spanned the width of the room, from waist to ceiling).

"I'm not looking so great," I thought.

I shrugged it off and then looked to my right. At that infamous full length mirror.

"Snap. That's worse than I thought," I shrugged.

The reflection gave me the first complete look of myself I'd seen *in over a decade.* As I surveyed my body, I noticed that I didn't quite look the same as I used to...

It's easy to deny reality, isn't it? I mean, I knew my clothes had been getting larger and larger, but somehow I *still* envisioned myself as the leaner, fit version of myself I was back in college. Sure, I knew I avoided pictures- or always pushed someone to stand in front of me and block my whole self from being captured on film- but I still envisioned myself looking sleek and svelt like I had in my younger days...

Full length mirrors don't lie, though.

My wife stood in our hotel room, just around the partition wall that separated the shower area from the rest of the room. She, too, prepared to attend the small event we'd been invited to with the company's founder. (It was her business success that won the trip. I was there as her guest!)

I asked her about my situation- in the form of a fishing statement. "I've gained a little bit of weight, haven't I?"

Now, *pause*. Before I go any further let me communicate to you that she'd gently tried to broach this subject with me for years. In fact, when I look back at our family pictures and vacation photos, the best I can discern is that I'd steadily gained 40 pounds in just over a decade of marriage...

That's just four pounds per year.

Only one pound every three months.

Or about 1/3 of a pound per month.

In other words, my weight gain was *virtually invisible* in the moment, but the compounding effect of bad food decisions (and removing most forms of consistent exercise from my routine) hadn't gone unnoticed. That incremental change, over time, was now obvious. *Extremely obvious.*

This wasn't the first conversation we'd had about this.

Somewhere along the third or fourth year into this trend, back when I was only 10 or 15 pounds overweight, she began asking me things like, "Hey- would you like to jump on the bathroom scale and see how things are going?"

Nope.

And, as she watched me chugging my beloved white chocolate mochas from Starbucks (with extra caramel drizzle and whipped cream, of course), "Do you think you might be *drinking* most of your calories?"

Drinking calories? Really? Who'd heard of such a thing? I thought you could only eat them.[2]

---

[2] Turns out, you can drink a lot of them. Last year I heard that the average male would lose 25-30 pounds in a year if he simply stopped consuming calories from drinks- including soft drinks, alcohol, sugary "sports" drinks, etc.. This is without any other diet or exercise adjustments.

A few months prior to standing before that mirror, my Mom and Dad sent me a birthday present. I opened the box to find a thermal running shirt. It was December, so the timing for this gift was great. I actually fancied myself as a pretty good athlete during this season (I know, laughable, particularly since I exercised for one 90-minute clip about once every 2-3 weeks). I remember unfolding the Nike shirt as I pulled it out of the box...

"It's an *EXTRA* large," I said. Then- "Why does my Mom think I wear a shirt this big?"

I'd worn medium shirts back in the day. Of course, back in the day I weighed 180 pounds. Now, I weighed about 220 (though I could peak as high as 225).

"Well," my wife replied. "It looks like it fits great. I think your mom did a good job picking that out for you..."

Anyway, these are the sorts of conversations that had peppered the previous six or seven years. So, when I asked her about my weight issues, *she'd already been trying to tell me for years. I'd just never been ready to hear it.*

So...

There, standing naked in front of a full length mirror, I asked, "I need to lose a few pounds, don't I?"

Drumroll...

"Yes. You could *stand to* lose a few pounds," she replied.

She was sweet. I could tell she didn't *really* want to be direct about it, because she didn't want to crush my pride. At the same time, though, she'd tried to communicate this for years. I'd finally given her an open invitation. So, that's how she phrased it: *I could stand to...*

"Like how much?" I asked. Then, I tried to quantify it before she could answer: "Maybe 10 pounds or so?"

She gave me a polite, sing-song *"Hmmm"* and suggested I move my number higher.

"15?!" I quickly responded.

"Ummm…"

"20 pounds?" I replied.

By now we were in the same room. She looked at me and smiled. She motioned that I should go to *another* higher number.

"*25?*" I asked, slightly elevating the pitch of my voice, to accentuate the five and the finality of the number. I knew I had *some* to lose, but her number was a bit higher than I actually thought…

She motioned a bit higher…

"30?"

"Yeah, probably so," she told me. "You could do at least twenty five…" (*At least?* I thought.) "…but probably closer to 30 would do it."

I started running the numbers in my head, thinking how impossible it would be to get to where I needed to be. How long it would take…

It was the end of February. I figured I was hovering about 215 or so…

If I lost 2-3 pounds per week I could cut about 10 per month, lose 35 by June and make it down to 180. I could achieve that before her birthday on June 1.

But was that even possible?

Big changes

I jumped into two things immediately upon boarding the plane from Hawaii back to the continental U.S. That's right- I didn't even wait until we got home.

First, I began helping her with her business. Up to this point, I'd been casually supportive, simply cheering her from the sidelines. I figured with some extra help and some extra time she could be even more successful.

That move eventually led to a transition from working outside of the home to working from home. Even though it's something I never thought I'd do, it's been one of the best decisions we've made. But, that's a longer story and a bigger topic for another time and place.

Second, I began losing that extra weight and getting healthy. Right now, I'm in better shape than I've ever been in my life. And, I've learned a lot about myself and health throughout this journey.

For instance, back when I was overweight, I couldn't sleep through the night. However, I could crash at any time during the time. Working 60-80 hours a week took its toll on me physically and emotionally. In the evening, I was too hyped on adrenaline to rest; during the day I was too tired to function. I found myself stress eating in order to simply cope. **Maybe you've been there- and realize that you, too, eat a lot even when you're not actually hungry.**

Another thing I learned was that I can't out-exercise a bad diet. Oddly enough, I was somewhat physically active during that season of life. I could run 5-7 miles at any time without stopping to rest (except I always walked big hills because of the extra weight). I even endured a few months of one of BeachBody's toughest workouts, P90X.

YOU CAN'T "OUT-EXERCISE" A BAD DIET

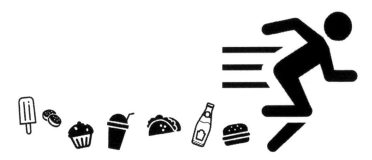

Despite the exercise, I found myself totally frustrated with my lack of results. I couldn't lose weight, regardless of how much time I spent sweating. So, I found myself consistently avoiding the scale, and my clothes continued getting both tighter and larger. My steady diet of sugar-laced Starbucks drinks, 2 pastries a day, and double-portion dinners created an environment in which health couldn't exist. Of course, you couldn't have told me that at the time, because my total caloric intake (in my mind) wasn't that extreme. As odd as it sounds, I even *regularly* skipped a few meals.

I learned that *eating* was the biggest factor in my weight loss- *not exercise*. That may fly against everything you've been taught, but think about it like this: a 7-mile run *may* burn 700 calories. One Venti white chocolate mocha from Starbucks on the way to work in the morning, and you've replenished all of those calories with junk fuel that adds weight to your body even though it's unusable for nutrition. Or one piece of cheesecake... that run is over plus you've consumed 300 *additional* calories.[3] Or one large lemonade from Chik-fil-A... you're better off

---

[3] Yes, get the nutrition info for one slice from the Cheesecake Factory and you'll see that my estimate here is actually a bit low!

snacking on a filet mignon than you are drinking their lemonade (and the diet version is worse for you than the "regular" version).[4]

Yeah, *the biggest factor was what I ate, not what I did...*

In other words, *both* diet and exercise are important. And it may be that the diet is *the* most important.[5]

The second shot of the year

Interestingly enough, the month *before* that Hawaii trip (January 2014), I actually entered a friendly "weight loss challenge" with two co-workers and a friend. Jon, David, Don, and I all agreed to a friendly contest. We'd *all* plumped up a bit.

The topic of our expanding waists came up one day after the first of the year while we were eating lunch at Overtime, a small dive about one mile from our office. Most people went there for the wings and burgers; I went there for the fried Oreo dessert. Topped with ice cream *and* whipped cream, of course.

(Disclaimer: I used to choose the restaurants I frequented based solely on their featured desserts!)

"Every morning we'll weigh in," Jon suggested. "Use your own scale. Take a pic of the number while you're standing there with nothing on."

---

[4] A large lemonade from Chik-fil-A has 340 calories- including 90g of carbs. Almost all of that is sugar- over 4x the daily recommended allowance on Keto. Plus, let's be honest, most of us get refills, right? A filet mignon has a similar number of calories- with no carbs.

[5] This is the first observation I make in chapter 12, where I discuss four big health issues I historically got backwards!

"Just be sure you don't capture anything else in the pic," David replied. "We only want to see the numbers on the scale."

We laughed.

Don suggested, "Let's put $100 each in the pot. After 30 days, the one who's lost the most weight takes all."

I actually thought I'd win the other guys' $300. Back in high school I wrestled. I could drop five pounds *in a day.*

Scratch that. Once I dropped five pounds *in less than three hours.*

It never dawned on me that I wasn't in high school anymore. Nor was I willing to starve for 2-3 days while layering up with sweat suits to drop the weight. I just thought, "Hmmm… challenge accepted. I'll feel good about taking $100 from each of you."

You know where this is going, because you know that the episode with the full length mirror in Hawaii happened *after* this. Yes, that challenge was about 6 weeks before my trip- the one where my wife told me about the "30 pounds or so" that I could "stand to" drop. So, you know that during this contest I didn't lose any weight at all.

I mean, I'd lose a few pounds in a few days and text it in: "Down over 10 pounds… all the way to 212."

Then I'd gain it all back. "Oops. I didn't eat as much yesterday but I'm up to 215 already."

I'd lose the same three pounds again…

Only to "find them" again over the weekend.

In the end, I actually *lost* the challenge. That is, not only did I have to give David my $100 (he crushed us all), but I was the one that lost *the fewest* pounds.

As I forked over the $100 bill I actually thought it must just be my lot in life to be a bit pudgy. I rationalized- and even told my wife several times- that "things change after you turn 40" and that I probably *couldn't* get in shape. After all, that was my experience during this challenge when I had a Franklin on the line, right?[6]

Counting calories, staying away from fat

So I failed miserably when competing with three friends. Then, I performed marvelously after speaking with my wife.

Dropping 35-plus pounds in just three months, my weight loss was noticeable. In fact, some people didn't even recognize me. Others who did wanted to know how it happened.

"You don't really want to know," I'd say.

"What do you mean?"

"There weren't any shortcuts. There weren't any quick fixes. I just ate less than I used to and I exercised every day. That's it. No magic bullet."

"What did you eat?"

That's generally when I told them about my spreadsheet. Although it didn't have "calories" listed on it, I had created an spreadsheet on my computer which had spaces where I entered data like:

- That morning's exercise routine

---

[6] Benjamin Franklin's face is on the $100 bill :-)

- How much I weighed afterwards (I stepped on the scale every morning before taking a shower and charted my progress)

- What I ate for breakfast

- Anything I had for a snack (I cut out most snacking, but wanted to record anything I even drank, due to learning that- *yes!- you can actually drink an absurd amount of calories*)

- What I ate for lunch

- What I ate for dinner

- Other notes about how I physically felt each day

I wrote *everything* down throughout the process. This turned out to be a great discipline, as it forced me to think about what I was doing. It caused me to make some "intelligent" decisions about my health.

And it provided me with options. For instance, some days I knew I was going to go out on a date with my wife (once every week). If we were going somewhere to eat that I really liked, and I knew I might want to "save calories" for that. I could adjust my intake earlier in the day and save it for later. Other days I was surprised at how much I had *already* eaten- or the fact that I hadn't eaten much at all yet.

Writing things down caused me to actually evaluate and think through what I was doing. This, to me, was as important as the diet and exercise.

By the way, I made a few predetermined decisions about the food I would eat over the next three months:

First, I decided not to skip any meals. My rationale for this was that when I was overweight I actually skipped meals regularly. I thought that would help me normalize my weight. However, I found myself ravenously hungry at the end of the day and would eat more in one meal than I would have all day if I'd just fed myself regularly. Plus, skipping meals caused my blood sugar to plummet, making me even hungrier (a problem you won't face on Keto, by the way).

It's actually shocking how many overweight people skip meals. I did. And I snacked. You're better off just eating a meal and not getting hungry for a "bad" snack.

Second, I made some decisions as to what I would eat for each meal. This kept me from making bad decisions in the moment. Honestly, I think this was such a key component of my success that I'll recommend this as one of your steps when I outline your path forward later in the book (chapter 15).

Here are some of the decisions I made about those meals:

- **Breakfast.** I decided I would eat a breakfast / cereal bar each morning for breakfast- and a meal replacement shake.[7] In hindsight, the cereal bars are one of the factors that worked *against* me. (More about this later.)

- **Lunch.** I ate a salad each day. You can get them anywhere you go- so it worked even when I had lunch appointments for work and was forced to eat at restaurants that you wouldn't typically consider to be healthy. I didn't have to worry about the breads that provide most of the calories on sandwiches (or the bloat and brain fog you feel after eating them), I didn't have to worry about fake vegetables from places like Cracker Barrel, and I didn't have to worry about explaining to their

---

[7] See the appendix. It doesn't work if you replace your meal with "junk" shakes.

people that I was on a diet. Every restaurant has salad, so it made things simple.

For sure, I had to be careful at some places (it seems like O'Charley's was the worst culprit), where some of their salads packed more clutter than what I considered to be unhealthy meals. Most of the time, I had steak or chicken on the salad. I've had salad at just about every restaurant in town- including all of the fast food places (which, oddly enough, have some of the best options).

- **Dinner.** I ate sensibly. I just ate whatever the family was having. The change-up here was that I no longer returned to the kitchen for seconds, thirds, or fourths. And I cut out the late night munching. Dinner was the final food I ate for the day.

Even without counting, I was still "counting" calories

That said, I lost the weight in 3 months. And I did it by "watching what I ate." In other words, I followed the traditional method of "stay away from foods that have fat in them, restrict your calories, exercise, and you'll make progress."

Here are two things I noticed, though:

First, over time, it became more difficult to lose the weight. It's almost like my body was "hanging on" to whatever I ate, refusing to let go. As a result, I found myself *exercising even more and eating even less* to lose the final 10 pounds.

NTRO- BEEN THERE, DONE THAT

It seemed like at some point I had to exercise in order to *just maintain* my weight. That is, the things that helped me progress in the early days of the journey didn't work in the latter days. I actually plateaued and "got stuck" a few times during my journey.

Second, I noticed that the calories I ate weren't "all created equal." That is, some foods seemed to "stick" with me a lot longer. Now, I'm not talking about candy bars and sugary drinks from the coffee shop- I gave those up on Day 1. There were other foods, though, that had a dramatic effect on how I felt...

For instance, most "health bars" and "energy bars" were junk.[8] I decided to eat those for breakfast everyday so that I wouldn't skip a meal. However, looking back, those bars did nothing more than create a short high followed by a quick crash.

Here's another one: drinking a sports drink (i.e., Powerade or Gatorade) left me feeling exactly like I'd just chugged a soda. Eating grapes actually made me hungrier, too.

(I'll talk more about why each of these things happened- and share some additional insights with you- later in the book.)

I eventually leveled out at my goal of about 180 pounds. But, as I neared 183 pounds, I began looking *sickish*. Some people even wondered if I was OK.

And I felt tired.

And I was hungry.

And that made me irritable.

---

8 I recently read the food label on one that I ate regularly during that seasons. Turns out, it has almost 50 carbs per bar! Sometimes, I would eat two in a day- before going on my weight loss kick.

The nameless sugar detox that excluded some vegetables & caused effortless weight loss

Just over a year after I lost the weight, my wife and I took a trip to Cancun- a second honeymoon of sorts. Her business had done quite well, so I turned in a two month notice and resigned from working outside the home. The day after my final day at the office, we boarded our plane and found ourselves in paradise.

There must be something about trips to far away beaches with my wife that causes me to start thinking about my health, though. A few days into the trip I noticed my tongue was coated with thick, white spots- a tell tale sign that I was ingesting way too much sugar.

Now, I wouldn't have characterized myself as a sugar-eater at this point. Back in the day when I was festively plump, *yes*. But now, *no way*. I generally skipped desserts, and I didn't grab candy bars at the gas station or pastries from the coffee shop any more. I hadn't tasted my beloved white chocolate mocha with extra caramel sauce in over a year....

Plus, for the most part, *I'd been hungry for the previous year.* I was thin, *but hungry.* And if I did indulge even just a bit, I doubled-down on exercise the next day or so and got things back in order.

As I stood before yet *another* double vanity in a beachside hotel in a faraway exotic location, I remembered a book I had sitting on the shelf back at home. Full of home remedies and go-to actions to naturally get your health in order, the authors said that the white spots on my tongue weren't just side effects of being a sugar-eater. Worse than that, they were symptoms of *candida*. That's right, *yeast*.

"Is it possible I have a yeast infection?" I asked my wife.

"It's possible," she said. "Maybe you should cut the sugar, anyway, if you really want to take charge of your health."

"What sugar?" I thought. Yeah, I'd eaten a few desserts on the trip. I'd tasted the "drink of the day" each morning when we hit the beach (yes, they start drinking alcohol *early* in Cancun). Those were exceptions to my normal eating patterns, but my tongue had been white for as long as I could think back...

I remembered a "test" the authors outlined in their book. "Spit in a glass of water," they said. "Does your blob of spit float or does it start growing these long, nasty tentacles from the spit blob down towards the bottom of the glass? Just wait a few minutes and see."

I grabbed a glass, filled it with water, and spat.

"What are you doing?" she asked. "That's disgusting."

"I'm self-diagnosing," I replied.

In less than 15 seconds long tentacles began growing towards the bottom of the glass- their "sure-fire" way to self-diagnosing *candida*.

"Looks like I might actually have a yeast infection," I concluded. "And not one of those that are located in one place in my body, but systemic... like throughout my body. When we get back home in a few days I'll follow the plan in their book and see if it gets results."

Now, before we go any farther, let's make an observation that may be *totally unrelated* to Keto. You probably have a book like that somewhere in your house, don't you? No, it's not necessarily a book about health. It may be a parenting book, a personal development resource, or even a tome about some skill you wanted to learn... yet it just sits there, even after a few years.

That's what happened here. About a year earlier I'd bought that book about detoxing and cleansing the body. "Life" got in the way, so I never got to it. In this moment, though, at the beach I remembered that the book contained that chapter on the effects of yeast on the body.

What's the biggest culprit? Yeah, *sugar*...

I decided to follow the plan written in the book and began detoxing sugar. That meant I followed a specific list of things the authors said I shouldn't eat...

- No potatoes (including baked potatoes, mashed potatoes, french fries, potato salad, etc.)

- No bread or bread-products (i.e., no sandwiches, no pancakes, no muffins, no bagels)

- No corn

- No bananas or strawberries

- No milk or cheese

Now, that's not the complete list, but **you'll notice something that seems strange about it: *there's nothing on that list I would have categorized as a sugar.***

About that time, too, I read William Davis' book *Wheat Belly.* The basic argument of his book is this: a huge amount of our health issues are caused by wheat- including brain fog, a long list of modern diseases that many people have simply learned to tolerate, and obesity. He writes,

"Aside from some extra fiber, eating two slices of whole wheat bread is really little different, and often worse, than drinking a can of sugar-sweetened soda or eating a sugary candy bar."[9]

The ills of gluten (which is found in wheat) have been in the press and pop culture enough lately that this was a no-brainer. Bread is (for the most part) bad.

But what about the other items on the list?

Were those really causing health issues in my body?

I jumped on the scales in Cancun. I wasn't afraid of them anymore. "180.5 pounds," I said. "Not bad, considering that I've been on vacation and have been eating like I'm on vacation…"

A few days later, after following the plan outlined for the sugar detox, I was at 174.5 pounds.

The following week I hit 172.

Then 169.5.

Eliminating sugar did something to my body that even exercise couldn't!

Furthermore, *I didn't feel weak or look gaunt* like I had as I hit the 183-ish pound mark. Remember, on that first diet I was simply watching my intake (read: counting calories without actually counting them). On this second diet **I actually evaluated the *kinds* of things I ate rather than the *volume* of things consumed.**

The name of that diet? I have no idea. All I know is that it forbade some things that I would have initially deemed as "healthy" choices, things I historically thought would help my weight loss. Turns out, I had a lot to learn…

---

[9] William Davis, *Wheat Belly*, p33.

And I began learning it *by experience*, one of the greatest teachers of all...

Your turn

Why do I tell you all of this? Well, if your weight has yo-yo'ed back and forth, if you've tried diets and failed, if you've tried diets and succeeded (but were left hungry), then I have a solution for you.

Over the next few pages **I'm going to tell you about the Keto diet- something that I enjoyed during that season even though I didn't realize what I was doing.** My promise to you is this:

- You'll lose weight fast

- You won't feel hungry

- You won't get tired

- You won't act irritable

Sounds too good to be true, doesn't it? I promise you, it's not.

Before telling you how to "do Keto" let me give you two assumptions. These will encourage and equip you as we take this journey together.

PART 1 | KETO BASICS

1. TWO ASSUMPTIONS ABOUT YOUR BODY

MAIN IDEA: ELIMINATE TOXINS + SHORE UP ANY DEFICIENCIES AND YOUR BODY HEALS ITSELF.

One of my friends named Dr. Jim Bob often says, "Health isn't easy, but it's simple."

Here's what he means by that. How to be healthy and live well isn't a secret. We know the ingredients of a healthy lifestyle. We've identified the nutrients we need and the environment that makes us feel alive. In other words, understanding the basics of health is *simple*.

That doesn't mean it's easy, though. There are a lot of decisions that need to be made- *and then lived*. Honestly, that's where most people miss it, in the follow through. We all know that we need to embrace certain food choices while rejecting others. We all know that we need a minimum amount of sleep each night or our bodies don't function as well. We all know we need to exercise in some way. Nonetheless, a lot of people don't do that either. Again, **health is simple- it's just not easy.**

In this chapter I want to show you just how simple health is. I'll do so by explaining two assumptions I have about our bodies. I promise, each of these has *everything* to do with Keto. In fact, **these two assumptions will provide you with a foundation for filtering the concepts presented throughout the remainder of the book:**

> • **Assumption 1:** *All dis-ease is caused by a toxin or a deficiency*
>
> • **Assumption 2:** *Your body is self-healing*

Now, let's make sure we grasp these two concepts before dissecting the basics of Keto in the following chapter. (We'll come back to these two assumptions throughout the book, evaluating what we're learning in light of them.)

Assumption 1: All dis-ease is caused by a toxin or a deficiency

Here's an easy equation you can remember:

High Nutrients + Less Toxins = Greater Health

The opposite is true as well:

Low Nutrients + More Toxins = Less Health

I know. That almost sounds too simple to be true, doesn't it? Here's why both equations work, though. Basically, all dis-ease in the body can be traced to two main causes: *toxins and deficiencies.*

What are toxins and what are deficiencies?

A toxin is something that *should not* be present in your body. Or, it's something that *can* be present, but it gets dangerous when it's present in too high of a quantity.

Toxins include things like sugar, synthetics, and even stress. Our body can handle *any* of these in small quantities, but too much can literally be lethal. As such, your body will generally *reject* them or *convert* them to a some other safer form.[10]

A deficiency, on the other hand, is when your body lacks something that *should* be present, when something that you need to support your body's systems isn't present in great enough quantity.

TWO CAUSES OF ALL DIS-EASE

	1. TOXICITY	2. DEFICIENCY
THIS MEANS >>	My body comes in contact with things that it does not need, things which are harmful to it	My body is not receiving some of the things it does need, things which would benefit it
EXAMPLES INCLUDE >>	Sugar, artificial sweeteners, cigarette smoke, high fructose corn syrup, gluten, etc. (stress is a factor here, too!)	Dehydration, lack of sleep / rest, calcium deficiency, exercise / movement
SOLUTIONS INCLUDE >>	Purity- eliminating toxins whenever possible	Supplement- flooding my body with nutrients and other things that boost my wellness

---

10 We'll see that sugar is a toxin. Your body's natural response? Get rid of it. Use as much of it as you possibly can as quickly as feasible and convert the rest to body fat.

For example, we need a certain amount of rest in order for our body's to recharge and recover. When that's missing, our body moves towards dis-ease. We also need specific nutrients and minerals. When we lack them... well... our bodies don't work like they're designed.

As you might imagine, there's an inverse relationship between toxins and nutrients. When one is high, the other is low. When one is low, the other is high:

- Higher levels of toxins = Greater level of deficiencies (*read: minimal nutrition*) = LOWER overall health

- Lower levels of toxins = Lower level of deficiencies (*read: nutrition*) = GREATER overall health

If I flood my body with the nutrients it needs, I'm not going to have many deficiencies. I'm likely not to have many toxins, either. For instance, if I eat healthy foods (nutrition up = deficiency down), I'm probably not eating that many unhealthy ones (toxin down). On the other hand, if I'm consistently managing too much stress (a toxin), I'm probably not going to get enough rest (thereby creating a deficiency).

Again, when we're walking in unhealthy patterns "the nutrient levels go down and the toxicity levels go up."[11] On the other hand, when we're experiencing health, it's because the nutrients have gone up and the toxins have gone down. We continue moving higher above the wellness line when we create an environment of nutrition.

(By the way, the more toxins you have in your body, the more fat your body needs to store them. This is why you can binge sugar for the

---

[11] Suzanne Somers, *Tox-Sick*, p127.

weekend have *instantly* feel like you have an extra layer of fat on your love handles or your thighs. More toxins present = more storage containers needed to handle the extra load.[12])

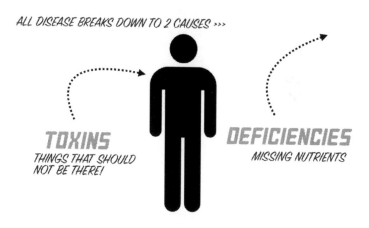

ALL DISEASE BREAKS DOWN TO 2 CAUSES >>>

TOXINS
THINGS THAT SHOULD NOT BE THERE!

DEFICIENCIES
MISSING NUTRIENTS

What does this first assumption have to do with Keto?

Well, if you're following the typical American diet, you've probably been steering clear of fats. You may be even eating "fat free," "diet," or "reduced calorie." Understand, I'm not belittling you- I did this myself.

Turns out, your body *needs* fat. It craves it. Lots of it. I never would have thought it to be true- especially in light of everything we hear in pop culture- but your body thrives on a high-fat diet. Most people- particularly overweight people- eat diets that are *deficient* in fat. They're missing nutrients that make the body work like it's supposed to. At the same time, they're filling the stomachs with "hidden" sugar- one of the most toxic things people can possibly eat (we'll discuss carbs in chapter

---

12 Suzanne Sommers, *Tox-Sick*, p154.

7). Put the two together, a deficiency and a toxin, and you have a recipe for disaster.

No worries if you're not convinced about this high-fat thing, by the way. I'll explain it in great detail in the next few chapters, as a fat-based diet is the cornerstone of the entire Keto experience.

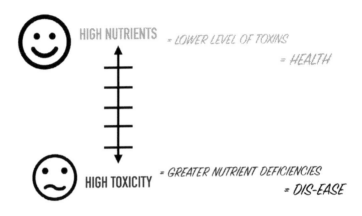

Assumption 2: Your body is self-healing

This leads me to the next foundational idea of the book: **your body is self-healing. That is, your body's natural state is actually health.**

This may sound contrary to popular opinion, too, because you don't have to bump into too many people on any given day until one of them will tell you, "My _____ [insert body part, major organ, etc.] has *never* worked. I always struggle with _____ [insert the related condition]." Some people say it as if it's a badge of worth or value that they have physical issues, that it's *not* normal to be healthy.

You may not *feel* healthy right now, but- I promise- your body's natural state is health. Remember, though, the foundational causes of all disease have to do with toxins (things that shouldn't be present) or deficiencies (things that need to be present). **When we remove the toxins and we shore up the deficiencies we create a body system that truly comes alive.**

MAKE IT SIMPLE!

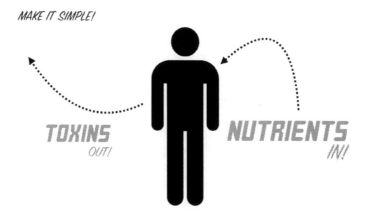

TOXINS
OUT!

NUTRIENTS
IN!

Most people practically forget things like...

- **Your body has an immune system**- 80% of which is housed in your gut. Your body *does not* have a disease system that manufactures illness.

  (By the way, this means that when we get our nutrition in order, we're serving 80% of our immune system at the same time. Now, you understand why junk food makes you feel like, well… *trash!*)

- **Your blood stream houses T-white blood cells, courageous fighters that literally war against dis-ease on your behalf.** When infection enters, they "call in" reinforcements and *multiply* in number.

  (One of the methods physicians use to tell if your body is fighting an infection is by counting the number of these warriors present in your blood stream. A higher number indicates that your body is waging battle against some unhealthy intruder. It's fighting for health!)

- **Your body automatically repairs itself.** Your bones will mend if broken (often healing more rigid than they were before the break), your skin will repair itself when cut, and your colon will expel food you eat that upsets the balance of your digestive system.

  (Yeah, think about that. Your body literally *fixes itself* when it becomes damaged!)

Now, all of this happens *on auto-pilot* every single day. You don't have to tell your body to heal itself, it just performs that way naturally. However, **when you provide your body with the best possible environment you can (one that is lower in toxins and has the nutrients in needs), your body becomes *extremely* efficient at optimizing health.** This is because when you create an environment in your body receives *more of what it needs and less of what it doesn't*, you actually create *better* space where your body can do what it *already* wants to do.

Putting it together

So what do these two concepts have to do with Keto?

Quite simply, this: most people come to Keto for the weight-loss benefits. I mean, let's be honest, the majority of people we know are struggling with their weight. After doing so for years, I just gave up and resigned myself to being a bit chubby.

Why?

- *Because losing weight seems difficult*

- *Because losing weight usually requires going hungry*

- *Because losing weight usually requires growing tired*

- *Because losing weight usually requires getting irritable*

That is, the cost seems too high. It often feels more beneficial to just keep things as they are, right?

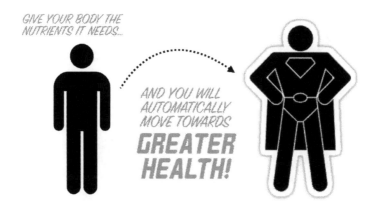

But, if health is actually simple…

- If health is a matter of "toxins out and nutrients in" like we discussed in the first assumption…

- If health is something your body actually *wants* to do…

… then moving towards your ideal weight shouldn't be a struggle, should it? I mean, if you provide your body with the right nutrients, it should happen *naturally*, shouldn't it?

Hippocrates, the father of modern medicine, said, "Let food be your medicine and let medicine be your food."

The first time I dropped the 40 pounds, there were days of struggle. Some nights, I was hungry. Because I charted everything I ate, I learned that some meals would cost me a small gain in body weight. That is, I'd go backwards from my goal. That caused me to develop a love-hate relationship with eating. I needed to eat to not be hungry or sluggish, but I was desperate to drop the weight…

YOU CAN EAT & STILL LOSE WEIGHT!

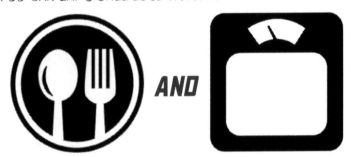

YOU DON'T HAVE TO CHOOSE BETWEEN HUNGER VS. WEIGHT LOSS GOALS!

You might have felt this way before, too. **You want to lose weight, but you don't want to choose between losing weight and starving.** If that's you, I've got some great news for you.

Later in this book I'll show you how the typical American diet of high-carbs actually hijacks your hunger hormones from working properly and actually makes you hungrier- even if you've already over-eaten. And I'll show you how the USDA recommendation actually cause your body to create and store more fat rather than eliminate it- all while making you even hungrier (see chapter 8).

You'll learn that the Keto diet actually works with your body's hormones to leave you feeling satisfied. Furthermore, Keto converts your body (and even your brain) into fat-burning machine!

Sounds too good to be true, doesn't it? *I promise you- it's not.*

You see, the Keto lifestyle takes Hippocrates' admonition seriously, realizing that the foods we eat can work *for* us instead of against us. That is, the foods you eat should actually *help* you lose weight such that you never find yourself in the position of deciding, "Do I stick with my weight loss goals or do I go hungry?"

In the next chapter I'll tell you how I found Keto. I'll outline a few of my initial hesitancies, and we'll see if this thing might work out for you too!

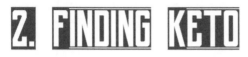 2. FINDING KETO

MAIN IDEA: LIKE MOST PEOPLE, I WAS SKEPTICAL ABOUT THE PROSPECT OF EATING A HIGH FAT DIET. BUT, YOU CAN'T ARGUE WITH RESULTS. AND WHEN I SAW THEM IN SOMEONE ELSE, I KNEW THIS COULD WORK FOR ME, TOO.

Two years ago, during the Fall, my wife told me she was going on a "new diet."

"I'm going to eat a lot of fats," she said. "And I'm not going to exercise as much."

Was she crazy?!

She read my nonverbal accurately and continued, "I was exercising too much. It was making me too tired to actually enjoy my day, so I'm going to look for something that works for me as far as that goes. And, I think my body needs more fats in order to actually function."

High fat. Low exercise. This was contrary to *everything* I knew to be true. I was sure she would "balloon up" over the next few weeks and then would make a more reasonable effort with something like "low fat" and "moderate exercise."

But something strange happened. Over the next few days- and I do mean *days*- I noticed her become more trim and toned. She continued eating a steady diet of things like eggs, guacamole, grilled chicken, and something called "bulletproof coffee."

Ahh, yes, bulletproof coffee. That's coffee with butter floating on the top of it. Kinda. Technically, it's coffee with about 2 tablespoons of MCT oil and two tablespoons of butter blended together. When created in a Magic Bullet or other small handheld blender the drink morphs into a cream latte-esque beverage with a frothy top that's superior to anything you can purchase at any coffee shop.

Bottom line is this: **she continued shedding pounds, and she wasn't exercising hard or starving to do it.** Or, more accurately, she wasn't exercising at all and she wasn't eating the typical "diet" types of foods.

I was intrigued. I began researching Keto online. I browsed through Apple Podcasts and found a few recordings to listen to while shuttling kids around town for things like volleyball and basketball. I ordered a few books from Amazon. Until someone in my family "went Keto" I really hadn't heard too much about it.

Here's what I uncovered:

> *"Ketosis is a metabolic state that happens when you consume a very low-carb, moderate-protein, **high-fat diet that causes your body to switch from using glucose as its primary fuel source to running on ketones…"***[13]

And-

> *"**Your body burns stored excess fat as fuel when you reduce your carb intake enough.** The healthy fats aid in the fat burning, increased metabolism, appetite control reduced*

---

[13] *Keto Clarity*, p32. Emphasis added. Note: glucose is sugar, ketones are fat.

*food cravings, energy, feelings of happiness, and clear
thinking."[14]*

The name Keto is short for "ketosis," which is derived from *ketones*.
Ketones are released as a byproduct when your body begins burning fat
for fuel.[15]

The short version is this: **when you "go Keto" your body shifts from
being a sugar-burner to being a fat-burner.** And, it doesn't matter if
the fat your body burns comes from the foods you eat that day or if it
comes from the foods you ate years ago that have been sitting "in
storage" as love handles, thunder thighs, or a bloated belly. Your body
begins melting away the fat.

What's the catch?

Here's the catch.

I know you're looking for the catch, because you're likely shuffling
through the same thoughts I was the first time my wife explained to me
what she was about to eat and not eat. "Having fat just melt off your
body sounds a bit far-fetched. That's not how things usually work."

You're right. That's not how it usually works. Generally, whatever we eat
goes straight to the hips, thighs, and gut, right?

---

[14] *Dr. Colbert's Keto Zone Diet*, p38.

[15] "Ketones themselves are produced when the body burns fat, and they're primary used as
an alternative fuel source when glucose isn't readily available…" See *Keto Clarity*, p32.

My grandmother had one of those country-looking wooden craft cutouts of a lady cooking in her kitchen. "A moment on the lips, a lifetime on the hips," it read.

That's what we expect. Eat or be thin. Choose one or the other. So, most of us choose *not* to starve. Yeah, given the options of being thin or "not thin" we'd prefer the first. But, more than that we prefer not to ramble around hungry.

Here's the deal. **Our bodies have a specific order in which they burn available nutrients.** Nutrients (in general) come in three forms: carbs, proteins, and fats. That's it. Just about everything you eat is going to be- and is going to perform- like one of those three. By the way, another name for each of these nutrients is *macros*.

HELPFUL DEFINITION

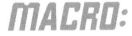 **"A SINGLE INSTRUCTION THAT EXPANDS AUTOMATICALLY INTO A LARGER SET OF INSTRUCTIONS TO PERFORM A PARTICULAR TASK."**

- OXFORD DICTIONARY

Before we go any further, let's define that word, *macro*. You may heard the term used before to denote "shortcuts" on your computer- something like typing in a few letters or command keys which results in your computer performing a complex set of tasks. That's actually a helpful way to understand what a *macro* is. The Oxford Dictionary says a macro is "a single instruction that expands automatically into a larger set of instructions to perform a particular task."[16]

On your computer, we call a *macro* a "shortcut."

As far as it relates to nutrients in your body, well... **there are three types of nutritional units your body can use.** Each of these *macros* **gives your body a specific set of instructions on what to do next.**

The three main macros are carbs, protein, and fats. Your body runs a different set of processes based on whatever each macro communicates to your body.

Here's a quick overview of the commands these macros dictate-

If you eat like the average American, the macro your body receives the most is most likely the "carb" macro. Carbs include sugar, starch, and fiber. Every carb you eat is literally one of those three. Fiber passes through your digestive system and isn't absorbed as a nutrient. It provides bulk to your stool and aids in digestion. Sugars and starches all convert to glucose in the bloodstream and are all treated by your body the same. That means that a Snickers bar (sugar), a banana (sugar), mashed potatoes (starch), and bread (sugar!) are all handled by your body in the exact same way. In other words, their macro gives your body *the same set of instructions as to what task to do next.*

That said, remember this:

- Carbs burn first. When they're present, your body runs their macro first.

- The body hangs onto the proteins it needs for vital functions, then converts the rest to carbs (this is all part of the "protein macro").

---

[16] https://en.oxforddictionaries.com/definition/us/macro

- Fat burns last.

In other words, if carbs are present anywhere in your blood stream, they're the first macro to run.

Ever heard the mantra that "carbs provide you with quick energy?"

Well, they do. *Kinda.* When they're present, your body cycles through what it can use. (And it stores the rest as body fat. We'll talk more about carbs in the upcoming chapter dedicated just to this macro, OK?)

Turns out, most carbs are starchy, sugary, and nutrient-poor. In general, they're not actually a great source of "fuel" for your body. In fact, many nutritionists believe that your body burns through them first in order to keep your blood sugar levels from getting too high- kind of as a "worst in, first out" type of response to the three macros that are available.

The fact that your body burns alcohol *before* it churns through any carbs is another argument in support of this theory. Think about it. A high level of alcohol in the blood stream can be toxic- lethal even. And, the same is true of sugar (a form of carbs). Your body goes into over-drive to eliminate the things that could, in high enough dosage, *destroy* it.

Remember that thing we learned a few pages ago about the "self-healing" body? And the presence of toxins and deficiencies? This *is that.*

Cashing out at the bank

By the way, any carbs that aren't immediately used for energy are stored on you as body fat. That is, they're stored in a non-lethal, non-toxic form where they can be used for "future energy use." In the same way that we put money in the bank for a rainy day, your body takes carbs and converts them to body fat stores for a potential time when you don't have access to food in sufficient quantities and need to, instead of eating, "cash out" those fat deposits.

Problem is, well... we have ample access to food. More specifically, we have ample access to an abundance of more carbs- more foods that our body converts to fat storage. In fact, statistics show that most of us *continue* banking and banking these fat stores *without ever making withdrawals.*

Furthermore, every time we place carbs in our system, we effectively tell our body to "get rid of them first." So, our body responds to the message and hangs on to the fat.[17]

My wife (the one who got me turned-on to Keto) explained to me, "If you eat fat instead of carbs, your metabolism converts. Your body actually craves fats. By not giving it carbs and creating a 'worst in' scenario, it begins burning through the fats you eat and the fats storied in your body."

A high-fat and low-carb diet effectively transforms your body from a sugar-burner into a fat-burner. The Keto eating pattern sends the message to your body, "Please use fat instead of carbs."[18]

Not only is this a completely normal metabolic state, your body actually *prefers* fats over carbs. In my reading I learned that newborn babies *thrive* on the ketones released from breast milk. They burn fat for fuel.

(This is one reason that babies who nurse tend to stretch out and get leaner while babies who drink formula tend to plump up. The formula is

---

[17] When you awaken after a long night's sleep your body has a higher ratio of ketones-because you haven't eaten carbs throughout the evening.

[18] See *The Ketogenic Diet*, p11.

loaded with carbs, causing those babies to burn some sugar and store the rest as body fat. I know, we're getting ahead of ourselves- we'll talk more about how this works in a few chapters.)

Now, I know what you might be thinking: "Yeah, babies suck their thumbs, they crawl, and they poop in their pants. Those are things adults shouldn't do. In fact, we hope babies grow out of that within the first year or so of life!"

I understand. You have some reservations. Like I did, you assume that this Keto thing might me yet another new fad diet, one of the latest crazes, something that will soon move over and make way to the next trendy thing.

So, let's go back in history. In the next chapter I'll show you the truth: Keto isn't new. Though it's seen a resurgence in popularity over the past year, the ketogenic approach to nutrition has been around for a really, really long time.

3. A QUICK KETO HISTORY

MAIN IDEA: THE HIGH-FAT-LOW-CARB EATING PLAN HAS BEEN AROUND FOR CENTURIES. IF YOU FOLLOW THE SIMPLE STEPS, YOU'LL GET THE SAME RESULTS THAT HAVE WORKED FOR HUNDREDS OF THOUSANDS OF PEOPLE IN ALL DIFFERENT CULTURES IN ALL DIFFERENT TIME PERIODS ALL AROUND THE WORLD.

Yes, Keto has seen a surge in popularity in the past few years. You can find podcasts about it, you read about it in magazines, and you see it in your social media news feed.

But Keto isn't new. In fact, you've got to go back a few *centuries* in order to locate its genesis.

If we travel back to France, there was a contemporary of Napoleon's who communicated some "novel ideas."[19] The year was 1825, just a few decades after the American Revolution and fresh off the heels of the War of 1812. Jean Brillant-Savarin, published *The Physiology of Taste*. **Two hundred years ago, for one of the first times in modern**

---

[19] Napoleon died in 1821.

history, someone printed that one of the main causes of obesity is starch in the diet.

Remember, starch is one of the three kinds of carbs- the other two being sugar and fiber. Moreover, his book stated that starch causes this weight gain "more prompt in its action" *specifically* "when it is mingled with sugar."[20] In one fell swoop, the Frenchman implicated both kinds of carbs that don't simply "pass through" your digestive system like fiber.[21]

He outlined a few tips as to how to avoid becoming obese: avoid white flour, don't eat dinner rolls, skip the biscuits, minimize your intake of all cake, stop eating pasta and macaroni, and never touch any form of potatoes ever again.

Sounds obvious, doesn't it? Especially when you remember that your body treats *all carbs* the same.

The man who became famous for treating medical issues with nutrition

Just a few decades after the Frenchman's discovery, an English undertaker (read: mortician and funeral director) named William Banting struggled to lose weight. Wealthy and obese, he spared no expense to get his health in check. After all, every single day he saw more and more corpses, and he knew his time was coming. He wanted to work on dead people- not become one.

---

20 *The Ketogenic Diet*, p14.

21 Fiber doesn't count towards your carb intake. It passes through your digestive tract. We'll discuss this more in chapters 6 & 7.

He followed the conventional wisdom of the day: "Cut your calories and start exercising more." But, rather than losing weight he continued gaining more and more.

If late night infomercials had existed back in that day, Banting would have been the first to hop on the bandwagon and buy *everything* from the Total Gym to the Abdomen-izer to Buns of Steel. He tried laxatives to poop the weight out, diuretics to eliminate bloating and water retention, and even- *get this*- starvation diets.

I know. You've probably tried some of these, too. I know I have.

Anyway, one day Banting visited a doctor named William Harvey in order to get his *hearing* problem treated.

"Let's treat it with nutrition," Harvey suggested.

Banting agreed. "Sure, but what do I eat?"

"Let's go low-carb," the doctor replied. "You can have a little bit of toast… some fruit… but not much of either of those. Let's focus on eating foods that are high in fat."[22]

You can imagine his initial reaction. After all, he'd tried virtually every imaginable way to lose weight already. And, even though he wasn't attempting to do that now, surely the doctor couldn't be serious about going "high-fat," right?

To his surprise, his ear issues cleared up. No more infections, and he could hear fine.

Then his knee pain got better. Turns out, carrying all that extra weight around had taxed his body and taken a toll. He hadn't even told the ear doc about that, but now his legs faired better, too.

---

[22] See some of his life story in *Dr. Colbert's Keto Zone Diet*, p17f.

Plus, he found himself having more energy than he'd ever had.

Oh, yeah... *he lost the weight that had burdened him for so long!*

In 1864, he wrote a book, *Letter on Corpulence, Addressed to the Public.*[23] He told of his journey into the world of nutritional health and how, by accident, he'd lost those unwanted pounds under the tutelage of Dr. Harvey. Furthermore, he reported that the *other* doctors' advice he'd strictly adhered to for years hadn't helped him lose any weight at all.

"Their cures were useless!" he said. He wrote that he "had been saved from a lifetime of obesity by the simple act of cutting out bread, sugar, beer, potatoes, and he wanted to do the good deed of sharing this highly effective, yet seemingly unknown, weight loss solution."[24] He outlined a diet that empowered him to drop over 40 pounds that year by restricting starches and sugars- just as the Frenchman had discovered a few hundred miles away.

Banting's book was an overnight success. This is remarkable, considering they didn't have Amazon or social media. Word still traveled quickly, though. In fact, the phrase *"Do you Bant?"* quickly became a euphemism for "eating a low-carb, high-fat diet."

Lessons from the wild frontier

In 1906 a Harvard-trained anthropologist named Vilhjalmur Stefanson traveled to the Arctic to live among the Inuit people for a year. He opted

---

[23] Download free here: https://archive.org/details/letteroncorpulen00bant, accessed 12-06-2017.

[24] *The Ketogenic Diet*, p15.

for a full-immersion experience, deciding to live exactly like them-
including eating only what they ate.

He quickly noticed a few things, all of which seemed *strange* to him:

- 75% of they calories they consumed came from fat.

- The lean pieces of meat were fed to their dogs.

- Vegetables were stored and saved for times of famine.

Remember, this happened in an area with incredibly cold weather, a
place you'd think people are more prone to feeling the rigors of the
weather. And, their diet- according to conventional wisdom- seemed
suspect. What seemed even stranger to him than all of this, though, was
that *he found no known health issues in the area.*[25]

Stefanson reported his findings and received mixed reviews. Many
people doubted that the diet the Inuit enjoyed was sustainable, even
though the Arctic natives had clearly been living that way for all of their
known history. So, in 1928, just over twenty years later, he and a
colleague actually checked themselves into a hospital in New York City.

"We'll just eat *only* meat and drink *only* water for an entire year," they
proposed.

They confidently believed they could prove to others that there was
something beneficial to the diet their Arctic friends ate.

The outcome won't surprise you in the least, particularly if you have any
bent towards natural health remedies at all. First of all, the medical
community protested. I know, no surprises there.

Second, those in the medical community who actually *wanted* to see the
results of the research and discover the truth- either way- finally caved

---

[25] *Dr. Colbert's Keto Zone Diet,* p178f.

to the pressure of their colleagues. Three weeks into the experiment, *the two were sent home.*

Of course, the experimenters didn't plan to give up. They continued the test on their own, communicating their results throughout their journey. After the year concluded, the men exhibited no deficiencies, had no blood pressure issues, showed no signs of hair loss, and demonstrated no discernible side effects. In other words, the low-carb-high-fat-diet proved sustainable.

Enter big pharma

Throughout the 1920s, family physicians prescribed low-carb-high-fat diets for epileptic patients- particularly for children. The evidence for this isn't just anecdotal (i.e., "I know of someone who knew of someone who...).[26] Far from it. Doctors at places as reputable as John Hopkins, Cornell, and the Mayo Clinic openly used this model of nutrition for their patients.[27]

In fact, in 1921, endocrinologist H. Rawle Geyelin stood before the American Medical Association at their annual convention.[28] (Your endocrine system is responsible for hormones and glands, and directly effects blood sugar levels, hormone secretion, and metabolism- all things we'll discuss later in this book.) During his presentation, Dr. Geyelin recounted his success in treating patients using ketogenic-

---

[26] Physicians today routinely shy away from anecdotal evidence. They want "science-based" findings.

[27] *Dr. Colbert's Keto Zone Diet*, p19.

[28] *Keto Clarity*, p206.

based nutrition. Then, he continued developing and refining his own version of the low-carb-high-fat plan of nutrition, a diet which became the medical standard of care until the 1940s.

During the 40s, though, a peculiar thing happened that prompted Americans to move *from* natural methods such as nutrition in order to deal with disease in their bodies...

Something that continues *even today.*

Namely, *pharmaceuticals.* For the first time, people could purchase a drug that treated the *symptoms* of the illness rather than having to address the deeper issue which was creating the symptoms in the first place. And, let's just be honest here, it's easier to pop a pill than it is to make a lifestyle change, right?

The (temporary) "death" of Keto

As nutrition began losing momentum as a legitimate method of health and healing because of the new availability of prescription drugs, *another factor* came into play that delivered the 1-2 punch. Enter Ancel Keys.

President Dwight Eisenhower suffered a heart attack, which threw heart disease- for the first time- into the public sphere.[29] Now, we talk about heart issues like they're commonplace (and they are). Until then, it was largely overlooked.

People everywhere began wondering, "What is this?"

Then, "What caused it to happen?"

---

[29] He was President from 1953 to 1961.

And, "Could this happen to me?"

A biologist at the University of Minnesota in the 1950s, Keys decided to answer the questions.[30] He believed there was correlation between fat intake and heart disease, so he launched two studies of multiple European countries to prove his theory.

This is an important point to remember: *he already had a theory he was seeking to prove.* Whereas the scientific method suggests the experimenter should make a hypothesis- that is, an educated guess- as to what they *think* the outcome might be and then run experiments that will disprove or prove that theory, Ancel went looking for evidence to back his pre-determined conclusion.

As a result, he looked for specific information *only,* and he manipulated the data to fit that theory. To be blunt, he buried info that didn't fit his model.[31] In 1999, over four decades after the original studies, the Italian researcher Alessandro Menotti (who happened to be one of the lead researchers for one of Keys' two studies) reanalyzed their data. He knew that original findings were skewed; he craved an accurate answer.

His conclusion was this: "sweets," not fats, were the greater influence on heart disease.[32]

That beckons the follow-up question: *Which foods are considered sweets?*

His answer: *anything that contains glucose.*[33]

---

[30] *Dr. Colbert's Keto Zone Diet,* p19f.

[31] *Bulletproof Diet,* p29.

[32] *Dr. Colbert's Keto Zone Diet,* p22.

[33] See Alessandro Menotti, "Food Intake Patterns and 25-Year Mortality from Coronary Heart Disease," *European Journal of Epidemiology* (July 1999), pp507-515.

And which foods contain glucose? Carbs. Specifically, sugars and starches (fibers aren't digested- they "pass through" your digestive tract).

In other words, Keys final reports revealed the *exact opposite* of what turned actually out to be true, according to his own original data.

Now, we can look back and assess what happened, but, the damage was already done:

- Fat was branded "bad"

- Carbs were "proven" healthy

- Despite what historical data had shown, low-fat-high-carb became the trend

The medical community rallied behind Keys. Food industries built around sugar, they began sponsoring lobbyists, and they targeted fat as Public Enemy #1. People's diets shifted rather quickly...

Food changes

With the high-carb kick in full swing, a few things happened to our food. In fact, a lot of food turned out *not to be food at all*. Here's what I mean.

First, in order to remove the fat from most foods and turn it into "low fat," you have to mechanically process the ingredients. So, "fat free" soon equated to "processed" foods.

(Most people agree that processed foods aren't healthy. Yet, in order to go "low fat" you must go processed.)

Second, fat provides the taste for most foods. Guacamole, whipped cream, and steak all taste great... in large part *because of the fat.* When you artificially remove the fat from foods, you not only turn the food into a non-food, you alter the taste in the process. In order to make the food palatable, you've got to add something back into the food (through a mechanistic process, of course) that puts some sort of taste into it so that people will actually eat it.

Here's an example: *milk.* People used to drink it "raw," that is, straight from the cow. The government decided raw milk isn't healthy, so a list of rules were created to govern how milk is processed.

Now, although you can purchase Whole, 2%, 1%, and even Skim milk at your local supermarket, *there are no such things as Whole, 2%, 1%, and Skim cows.* In order to get those variations of milk, the milk is taken from the cow, and run through a machine in a food plant. The machine removes the nutrients, allegedly kills the bacteria, puts chemically produced nutrients back into the milk, and then places it in a convenient carrying-size carton for you to place in your fridge.

Raw milk is high in fat, the fat providing most of the sweet taste. In order to make the processed milk taste right- so that you'll actually tolerate drinking it- the manufacturer has to add something back in place of the fat they extracted.

I'll give you a hint. They don't add protein into milk to create the taste. That leaves one option, carbs. That is, they add sugar into your milk. Milk off the shelf is loaded with sugar- as much as some candy bars.

Don't believe it? Go read the label on the carton in your fridge.

(The milk with the least amount of sugar is heavy whipping cream- it retains most of its fat and is a great Keto-friendly option!)

Third, fat actually makes you feel full. It *satiates* you. We'll talk more about how carbs hijack your hunger hormones in a future chapter. Suffice to say, when people aren't eating fat, they actually eat *more*.

(Ever looked at pics from the 1970s and thought, W*ow, everyone looks so... healthy? And everyone now looks so... obese?* Part of that is a lack of fat in our diets.)

Since there are only three types of macros, if you remove fat from your diet you're left with two options: protein or carbs (read: sugars and starches). Which one do you think people crave the most? Yeah... *sugar.*

Going "skinny"

Last weekend, Mini (my nickname for Miriam, our youngest daughter) and I made our monthly Costco run. We load up on the things we buy in bulk, then purchase fresh fruits and vegetables from other sources on a weekly basis. Mini had some shoes to swap from Vans, wanted to make a quick visit to the Lego Store, then make a pit stop at Starbucks. With 30 minutes to spare before retrieving the middle daughter (Ivey) from volleyball practice, I obliged.

"I'll take a grande caramel brûlée latte," the lady in front of me said. Then, as the barista entered her order into the touchscreen POS, "but make it a skinny one. It has to be low fat. I'm watching my weight."

"You're watching it go up on the scale," I thought to myself.

I know. Not a nice thought at all. But I was in the middle of researching this info about fats and sugars and since I frequent Starbucks I'd been looking at their nutrition facts.[34]

Here's what she just ordered:

- 270 calories (she was *drinking* more calories than the main course of a healthy meal)[35]

- 0g of fat (hence, the "skinny," even though this is the ingredient in the latte that could assure she won't stay fat)

- 59g of carbs (consisting of 44g of sugar and 15g of starch, thereby *tripling* with one drink the number of carbs she'd consume in a full day on a low-carb diet)

By the way, a latte has one shot of espresso with milk added to it. That is, her drink was mostly milk and flavored syrup.

Again, since our government agreed that "fat is bad," strict rules were legislated ousting raw milk from the supermarket. Now, all milk is processed. Milk suppliers take the raw milk, mechanically separate certain parts of it to ensure no bacteria or other harmful ingredients are present, and then add back specific nutrients. They also determine how much fat will be present in the final product (whole, 2%, skim, etc.). On Keto, you'll learn that heavy cream- the kind with the actual fat- is the best for you. Everything else has had a high percentage of the original fat removed and has carbs infused into the final product to enhance the hijacked taste. The "skinnier" the milk gets, the worse it becomes...

---

[34] Source: http://www.myfitnesspal.com/food/calories/starbucks-caramel-brulee-latte-skinny-18318192, accessed 01-11-2018.

[35] Yes, you can drink your calories!

Most "fat free" products are loaded with carbs- all of which your body metabolizes as a sugar because starches and sugars both convert into glucose.

Want to go sugar free and fat free? You'll have to add a synthetic instead. That means your body *can't* metabolize it. Yes, the calories still count (and add weight to you) but you receive *no nutritional benefit whatsoever*. And, "fake foods" (even fake sweeteners) hijack your hunger hormones and actually make you *hungrier*. (We'll talk more about this in chapter 8).

Again, the biggest source of funding for the anti-fat movement (including advertising, hiring lobbyists, etc.)... *the sugar companies*.

And that, my friend, leads us to where we are now. In the following chapter we'll talk about the actual data- and see what the actual historical facts reveal about Keto.

4. THE STRANGE THINGS CALLED FACTS & DATA

MAIN IDEA: THE LOW-FAT-HIGH-CARB DIET HAS BEEN PROMOTED FOR HALF A DECADE. AS SUCH, WE'VE HAD AMPLE TIME TO SEE THE RESULTS. TURNS OUT, THE LOW FAT MOVEMENT HAS BEEN A DISASTER.

Unless you've been living like a hermit, you've likely heard of the Atkins diet. Robert C. Atkins was an up-and-coming cardiologist in New York City in the 1960s. Young and intelligent, he was also overweight, lethargic, and had trouble managing his weight. Like William Banting virtually a century earlier, he too initially followed the wisdom of the day. After all, a heart doctor would want to avoid anything that might cause heart disease, right?

You know where this story is headed. Dr. Atkins got no results by following the low-fat-high-carb wisdom of the day, before stumbling upon a low-carb diet. Intrigued- and desperate- he took the leap. The results were instantaneous.

Since he was already a prominent doctor, people took notice:

- Companies hired him to consult their employees on health and nutrition.

- People throughout the country began following his new diet.

- Even *Vogue* magazine ran a story about his diet, which soon became referred to in pop culture as the "Vogue Diet."

Then the famous doctor published a book- a book that took the nation by storm.

In 1972, *Dr. Atkins' Diet Revolution* hit bookstores and news stands, and a mass audience was reintroduced to the high-fat-low-carb diet that had fallen from grace. Atkins explained the ketogenic metabolism in a way that everyone could understand and in doing so mainstreamed the idea of cutting the carbs.

(Note: there are differences between Atkins and Keto. I'll outline them in chapter 7.)

Here's where it gets interesting: In April 1973 a Harvard nutritionist testified before a Senate sub-committee that Atkins should be charged with malpractice. He *almost* had his license revoked.

Yes the medical establishment pressured the federal government to squash the Atkins revolution. However, word still spread...

The strange things called facts & data

Like I said earlier, Keys' research was skewed. It wouldn't stand to today's standards of research and reporting. Aside from our ability to look back and say, "Oh, he manipulated the data to support his pre-determined conclusion," we have almost half a century of data since transitioning to his suggested low-fat-high-carb eating plan. We can look at the fruit of following his conclusions and... well... the fruit doesn't taste too good.

First, let's look at the anecdotal evidence. Remember, anecdotal evidence isn't the kind of evidence we gather from strict observation in a lab. Rather, it's just what we notice when we look around, listen to people's stories, and observe what's happening in real life.

That said, think about it this way...

If eating fat makes you fat, then all of the people who are drinking those skinny lattes, choosing "fat free" foods, and choosing things labeled "diet" should all be thin, right? Or, at least, their weight should be going *down*.

But it's not. In fact, most of them will contend that they keep trying but that their body must be ultra-sensitive to *other* foods like fats (which they have to ingest in small quantities) and *that* is what's making them struggle. See the irony?

As well, if fat causes heart disease, then people who eat a low-fat-high-carb diets and regularly reach for foods that are labelled "low fat" should be safe from heart attacks, correct? Turns out they're the ones *having* the heart attacks.

Second, let's talk about the raw facts. The USDA and the FDA have now promoted Keys' low-fat-high-carb schema for almost half a century- all under the guise of preventing heart disease (something which was, in comparison to today's numbers, extremely rare 50 years ago).

We should see great results, then, shouldn't we? Again, we've had time to see the fruit of these decisions.

Heart disease was the original issue that sparked Ancel Keys to go after fat. Remember, he blamed fat as the culprit and pushed for the low-fat-high-carb alternative.

Today, heart disease kills 800,000 people per year in the United States alone. Claiming a new victim every 40 seconds, it accounts for 1 of every 3 deaths.[36] (Yeah, since you began this chapter, 2-3 people have died of heart disease.)

During the time our society has, for the most part, been abiding by these guidelines, *here's what else has escalated*:

- Obesity

- Type 2 diabetes

- Dementia

- Alzheimers

- High blood pressure

- ADD + ADHD

- Cancer

In other words, *the low fat movement has been a disaster.* Furthermore, "we now know from the research that sugars and refined carbs are the true causes of obesity and heart disease- not fats, we've been told."[37] *The Bulletproof Diet* reports that "An extensive analysis of 76 academic studies involving more than 600,000 participants found that saturated fat is *not* associated with coronary heart disease."[38] In other words, not only

---

[36] http://www.acc.org/latest-in-cardiology/ten-points-to-remember/2017/02/09/14/58/heart-disease-and-stroke-statistics-2017

[37] Mark Hyman, *Eat Fat, Get Thin*, p14.

[38] *Bulletproof Diet*, p45.

did Keys' lead researcher implicate another culprit in the heart disease issue (sugar), recent tests reveal that the case against fat should be dismissed.

My experience is that **most people who argue against a high-fat diet simply do so because they've *heard* that fats are bad.** Generally, they've heard it from a friend or from somewhere in the media. Most of them can't point to a single resource they've researched, something tangible where they've actually looked at the facts.

I'm not belittling them. Understand, I was in the same boat. When my wife told me she was going on a high-fat-low-carb diet I wasn't scared for her health; I just thought it wouldn't work.

Why? Because somewhere, once upon a time, I heard that fat was bad...

Turns out, though, that the research proves otherwise. I discovered:

> *"... ketogenic diets have been used to treat many conditions: infantile spasms, epilepsy, autism, brain tumors, Alzheimer's disease, Lou Gehrig's disease, depression, stroke, head trauma, Parkinson's disease, migraines, sleep disorders, schizophrenia, anxiety, ADHD, irritability, polycystic ovarian disease, irritable bowel syndrome, gastro-esophageal reflux, obesity, cardiovascular disease, acne, type-2 diabetes, tremors, respiratory failure, and virtually every neurological problem... also cancer and conditions where tissues need to recover after loss of oxygen."[39]*

Why show this list of conditions? Quite simply, you're probably reading this book because you want to lose weight (or maintain it), or you know someone who does. I want you to understand that you can do so

---

[39] *Dr. Colbert's Keto Zone Diet*, p54.

confidently knowing that you're not doing so at the expense of your overall health. The nutrition plan I'm about to show you helps with all of these other conditions, too.

(Again, think back to that concept we discussed earlier about toxins and deficiencies... and how your body "self heals" when you provide it with the nutrients it craves. Look at everything on the list. It is just a coincidence?)

And, remember, Keto isn't knew. Unlike other diets that have come and gone (and unlike the ones that will come and go) the high-fat-low-carb eating plan has been around for quite some time. If you follow the simple steps, you'll get the same results that have worked for hundreds of thousands of people in all different cultures in all different time periods all around the world.[40]

That said, let's move into the next chapter and talk about how this Keto-thing actually works!

---

40 In other words, "unlike many diet fads that come and go with very limited rates of long-term success, the ketogenic diet has been practiced for more than nine decades...and is based upon a solid understanding of physiology and nutrition science" (See https://www.DrAxe.com/keto-diet/keto-diet-foods-list/, accessed 12-07-2017).

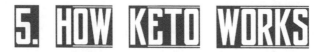 5. HOW KETO WORKS

MAIN IDEA: KETO SHIFTS YOUR BODY TO A FAT-BURNER INSTEAD OF A SUGAR-BURNER.

One of the basic premises of the ketogenic diet is this: *all calories aren't created equal.* In fact, that's the reason calorie counting diets don't work. You can stay below the recommended calorie threshold, but if they're the wrong kind of calories, you'll still gain weight.

Not convinced? *Think about it logically.*

Your body will respond differently if you eat two Krispy Kreme donuts for breakfast, lunch, and dinner than it will if you eat two small Filet Mignons for each meal. Even though these items both have approximately the same amount of calories, one option will leave you feeling hungrier and while the other actually satisfies you. Furthermore, you'll probably bloat (and may even gain a little weight) while eating the one but not the other.

I know, that's just hypothetical. So let's talk "real turkey."

The USDA presumes that the average male needs 2,000 calories / day for his basic nutritional needs. However, over the next few pages you'll see that saying "men need about 2,000 calories a day" is a bit too simplistic. It's like saying, "Every vehicle needs 10 gallons of gas to go 300 miles."

You and I both know that:

- Some cars need more than 10 gallons to go 300 miles- and some need less.

- The reasons why cars need more or less gas sometimes have to do with the car itself (i.e., larger cars usually need more gas, smaller cars usually require less), as well as factors outside of the car that can't be controlled by the car. That is, the terrain, the weather, and the road conditions can all affect the gas mileage. You'll get farther on the Interstate than you will in the city. You'll get farther on a smooth road than you will if you're driving through a rocky terrain or a desert.

- Different cars run better off different octanes of fuel. Some need high octane, some run better on low octane. Some don't need gas at all- they require diesel.

Knowing that, and knowing that the human body is far more complex than an automobile, it seems odd that the dietary guidelines published by our government presume that all people need the same amount of calories, doesn't it? Furthermore, later in the book you're going to be shocked when you discover what the kind of calories they prescribe for you actually do inside your body.

Car manufacturers know if they produce an inferior product, they'll go out of business. We'll move to the next company that makes what we need.

A predominant ketogenic expert observed that "If the USDA were a business and the state of public health reflected their profit margin, they would have gone bankrupt years ago."[41] In other words, **we don't hold**

---

[41] *Keto Clarity*, p10.

them to any actual standard of evidence-based proof. We just assume they know what they're talking about when it comes to nutrition.

The oddest think about following the government's nutrition advice is that we actually know that they don't offer the best recommendations in any other area. Think about it.

- Would you take budgeting advice from the government?

- Would you look to them for suggestions on how to *efficiently* run your business?

- What about parenting advice from the government?

- Or education?

- Take the example with which we began this chapter, automobiles. Would you even trust the government to coach you on the best way to service and maintain your car?

The answer on all of these is, "No. We don't think they have the best advice on any of this."

And, "We've seen firsthand that the government doesn't really do any of these things well."

In fact, the term "It's good enough for government" is synonymous with second-rate. We know that most things the government does don't get great results.

That's why it seems *so strange* that we all look at the nutrition guidelines published by our government- or at the catch phrases they toss out (i.e., "fat is bad")- and just indiscriminately agree, "Oh, OK... sure..."

What does the fuel do?

Back to the car. **Keto works by evaluating what the fuel you put in your body does as it passes through your digestive tract and into your blood stream.** It asks the question, "What do these macros do? What command do they run?"

Then, Keto makes decisions by tossing out the bad macros and putting in the good ones. The nutrition plan operates under the assumptions we listed in chapter 1:

- All health issues can be traced to toxins (too much of a bad thing) and deficiencies (not enough of a good thing), and

- Your body is self-healing

In other words, Keto creates an optimal environment in which your body system's can thrive. And, yes, **one of the symptoms of a healthy body is that you naturally shift towards your ideal weight**. However, there are numerous other benefits, as well.[42]

Over a decade ago my wife began shopping for our groceries at Whole Foods and some other healthier stores. As we ditched the cheap food at Walmart, I initially suffered from sticker shock.

"The grocery bill has gone up!" I noticed. I affectionately referred to Whole Foods as "Whole Paycheck," because that's what it seemed like they were taking from us- *all of it!*

"Yeah," my wife explained. "But it's better food. It actually helps your body."

---

[42] See chapter 14.

That's when I began to realize that most processed foods aren't foods at all. They're just fillers, edible food-looking products that are chock full of calories but void of any true nutritional value.

Over the next few months I noticed a few things:

First, their food did cost more but it lasted longer. When you're living paycheck-to-paycheck, it's tough to pay $5 for a loaf of nutritious bread when you can purchase Wonder Bread for $.99, right? Or a load of fresh vegetables when you can purchase entire meals for half the price.

Turns out, we ate a lot less once we began eating better food, because our bodies suddenly had fuel. Grasp that. *Your body doesn't just crave food; it craves nutrition.*

When you feel hunger pains, your stomach isn't saying, "Hey, just give me something to eat- anything."

Rather, it's communicating, "I need some good fuel. This body is running a million amazing processes all at once. We need something in the engine to keep this thing moving forward."

"EMPTY CALORIES" ADD WEIGHT EVEN THOUGH THEY HAVE

NO NUTRITIONAL VALUE

The dilemma is that *all* calories add weight to your body- whether they're healthy calories or unhealthy ones. Yet, again, calories are "not all created equal." Whereas calories from some foods are easy for your body to breakdown into nutritional fuel (you eat and find yourself satisfied), calories from other foods (especially the processed ones) aren't easily broken down. They tend to pack weight on, even as they leave you unsatisfied and hungry for more.[43] (Actually, some of the worst calories actually cause you to crave *even more* food!)

Second, our health actually elevated. To understand why, go back to the first of the two foundational assumptions. By eating better food, we removed toxins from our diet and we added nutrients. In doing so, we created an environment in which our body could "do its thing" more efficiently. (I know I keep repeating that concept, but it's super-important.)

Let me state something that's completely politically incorrect. Just an observation. Notice how many obese people are poor. You'd *think* they have less money, so they can afford less food, so they don't eat as much. As a result, you'd expect the poorest segment in the U.S. to be underweight.

Turns out, *they're not.* Their bodies are starving, but they're obese!

How so? *It's the kind of food they eat...*

How does this translate to our car analogy?

Well, I know it makes no mechanical sense at all, but my car actually runs better after I wash it. Yours probably does, too. It's almost like getting that little debris off the paint job (toxins) sends its spirit soaring.

The same thing happens whenever I change the oil (which, I know makes complete sense). Oil greases the system and allows things to

---

[43] Think back to the car analogy. If the car can't burn the gas, where does the gas go? In this instance, the gas just stays in the vehicle, increasing the load the vehicle has to carry, making it far more sluggish and far less efficient.

function. When grime gunks it up, things don't work as well. But, the transformation is almost instant, isn't it?

Third, in the long run, better food proved to less expensive than unhealthy food. Every time I mention this one, some math wizard grabs a pencil and starts pushing the numbers around to prove to my why purchasing more expensive food isn't cheaper.

Save the math. Here's what I experience firsthand every day:

We eat less, so the food cost becomes comparable. In the end, even though we pay more per sack of food, we actually require less sacks. We eat less, which ultimately costs us far less.

Or, to say it another way, "Yeah, the better gas is more expensive, but your car runs better and travels farther with the better fuel. In the long run, it costs you less."

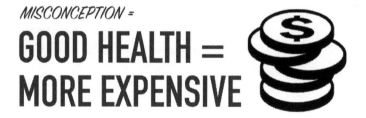

MISCONCEPTION =

GOOD HEALTH = MORE EXPENSIVE

We *rarely* get sick (because our bodies self-heal when they have the right stuff in them), so we never miss work. *How much do you think a sick day costs you?* Yeah, it costs you a day of wages, plus you fall behind on whatever you were doing the day before, whatever you were supposed to do that day, and whatever you were going to do the next day- all in the name of playing "catch up."

We also have more energy, so we enjoy our afternoons and evenings more. And, we don't use the weekends to recover from the physical drain of the week. Now, I know, you can't quantify that. But why do you have to? You see, better fuel is better for you.

To summarize, I learned this-

- **In the short term, you'll spend *about the same* on healthy food because you'll need far *less* of it**. It's nutrient-dense and actually works with your body.

- **In the long term, you'll spend far less on health, because *you'll avoid the costly issue*s associated with obesity and other forms of dis-ease**.[44]

How the fuel works in your body

There are two predominant fuel sources your body can use, glucose or fat. **Keto shifts your body to a fat-burner instead of a sugar-burner.**

---

[44] I struggled with referring to obesity as a dis-ease. Remember our definition, though: dis-ease is caused by deficiencies ("not enough" good things your body needs) or toxins (too much of something that it doesn't). Excess weight is something your body does not need; it's a toxin. In fact, the AMA has publicly recognized obesity as a disease. See the following:

- http://www.nytimes.com/2013/06/19/business/ama-recognizes-obesity-as-a-disease.html

- http://newsroom.heart.org/news/american-medical-association-says-obesity-is-a-disease

- http://www.npr.org/sections/health-shots/2013/06/19/193440570/ama-says-its-time-to-call-obesity-a-disease

That is, Keto creates a nutritional environment in which your body burns fat instead of glucose.

Your body is an incredible machine and can run off *either* of those nutrients. Just because it can doesn't mean it likes to, though. Nor does it treat them all the same. In the same way a vehicle responds differently to unique fuel source, so also does your body "run" the macros differently. **Our goal is to find the optimal fuel for your body, just as we like to do with our cars.**

Here's where it gets interesting-

Your body has the ability to run with different types of "engines." Your body can run as a:

- *Sugar-burning engine*

- *Fat-burning engine*

The only catch is that you've got to choose one or the other. You can't do both at the same time, and you can't efficiently toggle back and forth, either. In other words, even though your body works with either fuel source, you've got to make a decision as to which one you want to use as its "primary" tank.

Here's why-

- **First, any time glucose is present in your body it attempts to eliminate it.** It does so by converting it to immediate-use energy or by storing it for future use. Now, since your body has no way to store glucose in its present form, it quickly and efficiently converts it to fat stores.

- **Second, your body burns fat after churning through all available glucose.** Fat is the "last resort."

This doesn't mean that fat is the least preferred fuel. Rather, fat is the least toxic. Remember, your body works on a "worst-in-first-out" (WIFO) type of grid. Since glucose (read: sugar) is more toxic than fat, your body deals with it first.

I used to wonder how guys that drank lots of beer grew those huge "beer bellies." You've seen them, I know. Here's how it happens...

First, though alcohol itself contains very few calories, the delivery mechanism for alcohol always contains numerous calories in the form of carbs.[45] Hard liquor generally has the least amount of carbs, wine has a medium amount of carbs, and beer is loaded with carbs (read: sugar).

When you drink beer, your body senses the carbs and automatically begins running the macros. Remember, the macros issue "long form" commands as to what your body should do with each of these nutrients.

HOW TO GET A BEER BELLY

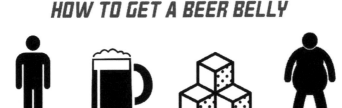

YOU + OVER-INDULGE = SUGAR STORED = RESULT

Since alcohol is more lethal than sugar, your body begins eliminating the alcohol before the sugar (WIFO). Even though your body is busy

---

45 I can't tell you how many times people have argued with me about this at the gym! Alcohol has 7 calories per gram, which is higher than carbs and protein, but most alcoholic drinks have very little actual alcohol in them.

focusing on the alcohol problem, it still has to handle the sugar, though, lest your blood sugar levels become too high. So, it "macros" the extra sugar like it always does and stores it as fat.

The previous graphic makes it crystal clear.

Now, I know you didn't read this book to learn how to grow a gut. Chances you are, you're trying to get rid of a belly, some of your bottom, extra weight on your thighs, or some part of your hips. No worries. I've got you covered.

I gave you the previous example to explain this: drinking a lot of alcohol creates a scenario where you can gain weight faster, but eating extra sugar *of any kind* does the trick just as well.

You see, when you run the sugar-burning engine option, your body uses what it needs for immediate energy, and then stores the rest. Your muscles hold about 1,600 calories of glycogen (water-based glucose). This will supply your body with about a day worth of energy storage. Your body will continually "top off" these reserves when you eat sugar. But, since most of us never completely deplete them before eating another meal, your body automatically converts the rest of the sugar to body fat.

On the other hand, **if you run the fat-burning option, your body uses the supply of fat you already have on hand as its primary fuel source. Nothing is stored as glycogen; nothing is stored as body fat.** As a result, "muscles and most other tissues stop taking in glucose for energy and start using fat instead."[46] This means that your body fat starts melting away.

This makes you wonder, then, how much fat do you have in storage? How much can be used? Well, one author writes,

---

[46] *The Ketogenic Diet,* p78.

"Unlike fat stores, which have over 130,000 [calories]-theoretically enough to last for months- glycogen holds only 1,600 [calories] and is depleted in about a day. When all the glycogen has been depleted, the body turns to its fat cells as an energy source and, as long as you don't eat carbs, ketosis sets in."[47]

To lose one pound you've got to "burn off" 3,500 calories more than you eat. That means the average adult has about 37 pounds of fat waiting to be used.

Sounds like a lot, doesn't it?

A few months ago I decided to test the theory myself. I take my oldest girls out on a "date night" the first Thursday of every month. It's a standing commitment written into our calendars I intend to keep until they marry. Then, who knows, maybe their mom and I will join them and their spouses.

The first Thursday evening of February, Ivey's volleyball practice went long, so we got a late start. We ate dinner, went to the coffee shop, and then decided to catch a late movie. I saw the "start time" for the film, factored how long previews would take, and estimated I wouldn't get home until 1:30 am that night. That meant I probably wouldn't make my 6:00 am gym time.

"Forget about it," I thought. "Emma is 17 and will only be in the house for about 18 more months. That means I've only got a handful of these nights left. I'll catch up at the gym another day."

Then it dawned on me, though. I'd been wondering how well the Keto diet worked *without exercising*. Every other time I'd tried the diet, I'd been running 5-7 miles a day (longer on the weekends) or doing high

---

[47] The Ketogenic Diet, p79.

intensity interval training 5-6 days a week. It's easy to lose weight when you've got that kind of output.

What if you removed that kind of calorie burn, though? Could I still lose weight? Furthermore, could I lose weight when I was already in great shape, seemingly not having much weight to lose to begin with?

This would provide the perfect opportunity for me to "test drive" Keto without exercise. And that would let me see how much of the "fitness" was the exercise regimen I kept and how much was actually the diet.

Here's what happened.

When I began, I weighed about 180 (since losing the bulk of my weight a few years ago, I hover around 180). Four weeks later, I weighed 165. Now, I don't have 37 pounds of fat to lose. In that sense, I'm significantly "below average." But, I clearly got into a position in which I actually needed to eat more and put some weight back on!

Clearly, my body made the shift- again- and learned to burn fats instead of carbs.

How you can make the shift, too

I know, you're wondering, *how do I make this shift and begin using the fat-burning engine instead of the sugar-burning engine?!*

In order to shift tanks you've got to do two things:

- **First, you must deplete your body of all of the "gas" (read: carbs / glucose) currently in your system.** This is easy to do, because your body's default mode is to burn these first when they're present.

- **Second, you've got to commit to the shift.** You cannot "mix fuels." Remember, whenever they're present, carbs will burn first. So, if you have both of these macros inside your body, you'll shift to the sugar-burning engine. In order to continue burning fat you need to keep the carbs out (other than the minimal amount we'll discuss later).

(By the way, I'll give you more specific tips about getting started on Keto in chapter 15.)

This second point above means *no cheat days.* I've never understood cheat days anyway. When I did my initial 40 pound weight cut, I didn't want to take a cheat day. I knew that if I did I would forfeit that day's gains, I'd reverse the previous day's, and I would have to start over the following day. In effect, one cheat day- even a cheat meal- cost me three days of progress. Frankly, I was making too much progress (and I was working too hard at it), so I decided it wasn't worth it.

ONE OR THE OTHER?

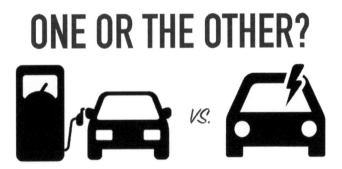

YOU CAN BURN SUGAR OR FAT, BUT YOU CAN'T DO BOTH AT THE SAME TIME.

When you're in the "fat burning mode," you definitely don't want to cheat. If you do, a few things will happen:

- **You'll "switch engines" and reset your fuel source to carbs.** That means you'll have to start over, eliminating all the carbs from your body and swapping back to "fat-burning mode."

- **Your cravings will shift.** You'll find that your body actually craves more of whatever it eats. When you're eating fats, your body begins craving them as the preferred fuel source. On the other hand, when you're eating carbs, well... your hunger hormones actually hijack your digestive system (we'll cover this in depth in chapter 8).

My point-of-view is that it's not worth cheating. Once you start making progress towards your weight loss goal, and once you experience the other benefits of ketosis, you're going to want to remain in that sweet spot. (By the way, **most Keto "insiders" refer to fat-burning mode as "being in ketosis."**)

Once you make the switch into ketosis, your body will burn the fat you eat and the existing fat storage you have. As a result, you *won't* feel hungry, because hunger is your body's way of telling you, "Hey, we need fuel." If you're average, you've got about 37 pounds of fuel- much of it available for use.[48]

Should you lose all of that storage? Absolutely not. But, Keto allows you to tap into the storage that you need to lose.

Now, every few weeks someone approaches me with the argument, "I'm big boned."

Or, "I have fat genes."

---

[48] The average 145-pound male has 135,0000 cal stored. 3,500 calories per pound is approximately 37 pounds (3,500 calories / pound x 37 pound s= 129,500 calories ready to burn).

Let me break it down for you. *Neither one of those is a medical condition.* I would encourage you to simply write down what you eat for a week without making any changes. Take a close look at the macros in each of those foods (I'll teach you how to read labels in the next chapter). My guess is that you're eating foods- lots of glucose- that cause inflammation (read: swelling, puffiness).

Your best bet?

Don't take the government's advice on your health. We don't trust them to handle any other personal issues for us, do we? Whereas that government is far more equipped than we are to handle defense, public utilities, civil services like fire and safety, you're better equipped to handle *you*.

Don't make a purely economic decision, either. Financially cheaper food always comes with a much higher non-financial cost in the short run, followed by an even greater financial investment at some point in the future.

Rather, **look at what the macros do. Then make the shift.** Swap from running your body on glucose and begin running your system on fats.

Need more info? In the next chapter I'll break down the three main macros for you.

6. THREE TYPES OF FUEL YOUR BODY USES

MAIN IDEA: A MACRO IS KIND OF NUTRITION THAT GIVES YOUR BODY INSTRUCTIONS ON WHAT TO DO WITH THAT SPECIFIC SOURCE OF FUEL. YOUR BODY CONSISTENTLY FOLLOWS THE SAME PROTOCOL FOR EACH MACRO.

Earlier in the book I introduced you to the concept of macros. When "computer guys" talk about macros, they refer to shorthand commands that your machine quickly translates and expands into a longer form set of instructions. A macro saves time, because you don't have to explain- in long form- what to do every time the same situation presents itself.

Nutritionists refer to macros a little bit differently. Rather than defining what a macro *does* (which is the most important fact about the macro), they most often tell us what the macros are. For example:

> "So what are macronutrients exactly? Plain and simple, macronutrients are the three categories of nutrients you eat

most and provide you with most of your energy: protein, carbohydrates, and fats."[49]

Or, look at this one:

"What is aware eating? It's knowing what your food is made of, and using that information to eat better. One of the best ways to do that is to start by tracking the macronutrients—protein, carbohydrates, and fats; as well as total calories—that make up what you already eat."[50]

See what I'm saying? **Nutrition sources tell us the kind of macros we find in foods, but they don't tell us the most important aspect of them, *what the macros do.***

So let's go back to the computer world. There, a macro is a "shorthand command." Once received by the operating system, the computer automatically runs predetermined processes.

The same thing happens in your body. There are five (not three) macros. Each one gives your body a specific command of what to do with that bit of nutrition. And, sure enough, your body does the exact same thing with each different kind of macro every single time.

There's no guesswork. **This means that since you know how your body will respond, you know the commands to give. That is, you know what foods to eat, because you already know what your body will do with each one.**

---

49 http://www.cookinglight.com/eating-smart/macro-diet-counting-macros-weight-loss-better-nutrition

50 https://www.bodybuilding.com/content/from-here-to-macros-4-steps-to-better-nutrition.html

Learn all five macros, then focus on three

Most sources refer to three macros only:

- Carbs

- Protein

- Fats

We'll discuss each of these throughout this book, as there the three you'll find in most nutrition books, food apps, and prepackaged labels.

I want you to be aware, though, of the following two *additional* macros:

- Alcohol

- Ketones

We discussed alcohol briefly in the previous chapter. You may remember that alcohol has "no essential function in the body."[51] In other words, it's not needed (i.e., "not essential") and it provides no nutrition. It's *empty*.

Most alcoholic drinks contain no more than just a few ounces of actual alcohol (alcohol has 7 calories per gram). As such, the delivery mechanism for alcohol is its nutritional pitfall, as its usually *loaded* with carbs (in the form of sugar, sugar, and more sugar).

We haven't discussed ketones that much to this point. Ketones are the by-product that's released when your body runs off fats. They'll appear in your blood stream, which makes a quick blood test one of the best ways to see if you're "in ketosis" or not.

---

51 *The Ketogenic Diet*, p76.

Since Keto has become one of the "latest and greatest" diet fads (even though it's not new), a lot of supplement manufacturers have started producing pills that have ketones in them. They contend that you can ingest their supplement and thereby raise the levels of ketones in your bloodstream, thereby proving that you're in ketosis and are burning fats.

That's putting the cart before the horse, though. The true measure of ketosis *is not whether or not you have ketones in your blood.* That's simply a symptom of ketosis. Rather, the true measure of ketosis is whether or not your body burns fat for fuel or burns glucose.

If you artificially add ketones to your bloodstream (by taking a supplement that raises your level), you'll receive an artificially high reading. In other words, you may "show" that you're in ketosis even if you're not.

The best option? Eat right and spend your "supplements" money on something else, something that aids in digestion or provides other items your body needs.[52] Your body creates ketones every day anyway, using them to provide a small amount of energy (mainly to your brain and your nervous system). Your body will naturally step up production and create *even more* ketones by itself when carbs aren't present and you're in the zone. At that point, they'll become a more significant source of energy.

Let me remind you that ketones, oddly enough, are "not essential."[53] You can make all you need. Your body generates ketones from fat in your body, as the fat is broken down.

That said, let's go back to the three main macros. We'll keep our overview short + sweet in this chapter, as I've dedicated an entire

---

[52] See chapter C. in the back of the book for a complete run down on what I actually use and recommend.

[53] If something is "essential," it means your body doesn't produce it naturally. That is, you must ingest it in order to get it.

6. THREE TYPES OF FUEL YOUR BODY USES

chapter to each of these individually. (We'll discuss carbs in chapter 7, protein in chapter 9, and fats in chapter 11.)

Basic facts re: the three main macros

There are a few things I want you to notice about the three main macros, so let's look at them side-by-side.

First, the calorie count. If you're calorie counting *only*, you'll likely veer in the wrong direction.

Notice that fat is the most dense nutrient. This initially causes dieters to second guess it. After all, if you're strictly calorie counting, your goal automatically becomes to eat less calories *in any form,* right?

Not so fast. Remember, **the calorie count reveals the amount of fuel in the food. The calorie count is not a macro. Therefore, it tell us nothing about how the body handles the calorie once it hits your bloodstream. That's decided by *the kind* of nutrition it is, *not the amount* of nutrition.** Again, don't be fooled by the calories. It's not the amount of fuel you use (only), it's the kind of fuel.

Second, what's *not* written on the food labels. I've provided you with the three macros here, because the kind of macro the food is dictates what happens when you eat it. Two of these macros contain multiple categories.

A protein is always a protein is always a protein is always a protein. Period.

But there are three kinds of carbs. Carbs consist of sugars, starches, and fibers. Your body responds to sugars and starches the same way.

This means that mashed potatoes (starch) and bananas (sugar) and Snickers bars (sugar) run the same "program" in your body. (Fiber provides heft to your stool and is eliminated.) There are also multiple kinds of fats. For the sake of simplicity, I'll punt that issue until chapter 11.

Third, finally, the grams. Nutrition labels count food in grams. Not pounds. Not ounces. Not servings. Not packages. *Just grams.*

The result of this is that when you begin tracking your intake (easy to do if you use a smartphone app), you'll want to evaluate based on grams. No worries, this is super simple to do. By now, most apps have determined how many grams are in a package, a piece, or a product.

On the following page I've created a chart to give you an overview. Familiarize yourself with it, because we'll continue adding information to this over the next few chapters.

From the "notes" on protein in the chart you'll notice this: **protein is not a significant source of energy.** Protein is used by your body to repair muscle tissue (and is part of your bone structure), and it's used to catalyze various reactions in the body. The body primarily conserves protein rather than using it for energy, since it's vital for so many important functions. This is important to remember, because a lot of people think that if you don't eat protein in large quantities that you won't have any energy.

Now, look at the three macros. Your body primarily uses glucose (carbs) or fats for energy.

THREE MACROS

	CALORIES / GRAM	NOTES
CARBS	4	The first macro your body will burn. These convert to glucose in the blood, promoting your body to act as a "sugar-burner." Sugars, starches, and fibers are the three carbs. Fiber is eliminated, so the grams you eat of fiber do *not* count towards your carb count.
PROTEIN	4	Protein is used by your body to repair muscle tissue, as well as to catalyze various reactions in the body. The body primarily conserves protein rather than using it for energy, since it's vital for so many important functions.
FATS	9	Fats are the cornerstone of Keto. They're the most nutrient-dense macro. Eating fats moves your body into ketosis, whereby your body becomes a fat-burning machine.

By the way, any overage of protein that you consume converts to glucose and is treated like a sugar. We'll talk more about this in chapter 9. For now, though, I mention it so that you see that **there are two primary sources of fuel you need to consume, protein and fats.** The other macros we mentioned briefly are non essential, that is, you don't have to eat them in order for your body to run extremely well.[54]

---

[54] You read that right. You don't have to eat carbs, alcohol, or ketones. Here's why: ketones are produced naturally as fat is broken down in the body. Alcohol has no essential function and always comes with a excessive number of carbs. Finally, carbs aren't required. Your body can generate all the energy you need from fat. Plus, extra protein is converted to glucose (which is what carbs convert to). Problem solved.

Learn to read your labels

All that said, in order to navigate Keto you'll need to start reading food labels. Though they look intimidating, they're super easy once you know what you're looking for *and what doesn't matter.* (If this sounds repetitious, bear with me.)

Here's where to begin: **first, look for the macros-** *not the calories.* Again, it's not just the amount of fuel that's important, it's the kind of fuel that's even more important.

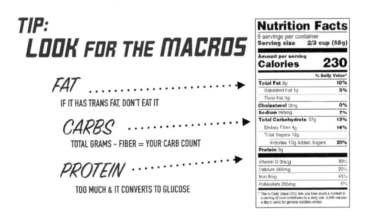

(By the way, all prepackaged foods and drinks are required by law to provide you with a nutrition label. I pulled the sample label below from the USDA's website. All labels will look similar to this one.[55] As well,

---

[55] Accessed on 12-06-017: https://health.howstuffworks.com/wellness/food-nutrition/facts/how-nutrition-works7.htm

most restaurants have the info readily available on their websites. And, there are dozens of great apps that provide you with this info, as well.[56])

Second, **look at the gram count for each of the macros**. For some macros this is easy. For instance, protein is super simple. However, for other macros this proves a bit difficult.

Take a look at the carbohydrate count on this label, for instance. We see that each serving contains the following:

- 37g of total carbs

- 4g of dietary fiber

- 12g of total sugars (the added sugars number is irrelevant info for us, as we're concerned with the *total* amount of sugar, regardless of where it originated)

Notice anything strange? Yeah. We have the total carb count, but we don't have info on each of the three kinds of carbs. For some strange reason, the USDA decided starches didn't need to be included on the labels.

TIP:
CARBS TO BE CONCERNED ABOUT

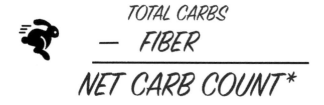

$$\begin{array}{r} TOTAL\ CARBS \\ -\ FIBER \\ \hline NET\ CARB\ COUNT* \end{array}$$

* FIBER DOESN'T COUNT TOWARDS CARB INTAKE B/C IT'S NOT DIGESTED. IT'S ELIMINATED!

---

[56] I use the *Lose It!* app.

We can do the math ourselves, though. This product contains 21g of starch (37g total carbs *minus* 4g fiber *minus* 12g sugar = 21g unaccounted for).

Why doesn't the label include starch? Honestly, have no idea. Just remember that starches are carbs. As such, they tell your body to run the command for that macro. They treat the starch like it's a sugar.

By the way, the FDA announced their rationale for the new labels:

> *"On May 20, 2016, the FDA announced the new Nutrition Facts label for packaged foods to reflect new scientific information, including the link between diet and chronic diseases such as obesity and heart disease. The new label will make it easier for consumers to make better informed food choices. "*[57]

That info comes straight from their website. Remember, though, we can't blindly assume that FDA's guidelines will work. They're assuming saturated fat is the culprit behind heart disease, and they're not counting starches towards carbs. "New" scientific information, as the FDA reportedly uses, would look back at the previous 50 years and say, "Hey, wait! The evidence doesn't show the correlation between high fat and heart disease that we once thought it did."

Ratios for Keto

Now that you know have an understanding of how to read the labels, let's discuss the ratios of these macros that your body needs in order to consistently burn fat.

---

[57] Accessed on 12-06-2017: https://www.fda.gov/Food/GuidanceRegulation/ GuidanceDocumentsRegulatoryInformation/LabelingNutrition/ucm385663.htm.

Throughout the remainder of the book, I assume 2,000 calories as our daily basis. Just understand that some people need more calories and some people need fewer. **And on Keto, you don't really count calories- you just eat when you're actually hungry.** Regardless of the calories, though, the ratios remain the same.

On the Keto plan, you eat with a "four-to-one ratio of fat to combined protein and carbohydrate."[58] This means 80% of your intake is fat; 20% is everything else.

If on a 2,000 calorie per day intake:

- 80% of your nutrition will come from FATS (1,600 calories, 178g)

- 15% of your nutrition will come from PROTEIN (300 calories, 75g)

- 5% of your nutrition will come from CARBS (100 calories, 25g)

Again, notice that "very few of your calories come from carbohydrates, a small portion come from protein, and the majority come from fat."[59]

I've done the math for you to provide you with the approximate number of grams you'll of each macro each day. Fats have 9 calories per gram, so we ingest just under 180 grams of fat each day (1,600 calories / 9 calories per gram = 177.78 grams). Protein and carbs both have 4 calories per gram. This means we eat 75 grams of protein (300 / 4 = 75) and 25 grams of carbs (100 / 4 = 25).

Most Keto experts will tell you to stay in the 20-30 gram range in order to stay in ketosis. This puts us right in the middle of the pack.

---

[58] *Keto Clarity*, p31.

[59] *The Ketogenic Diet*, p13.

Here's a look at the ratios on a chart.

TARGET RATIOS, ASSUMING 2,000 CALORIES/DAY

	% OF DIET	CALORIES	GRAMS
FATS	80%	1,600	178
PROTEIN	15%	300	75
CARBS	5%	100	25

And here's the pie chart view to compare caloric intake with grams. You'll notice that the percentage of fat calories seems drastically high on Keto.

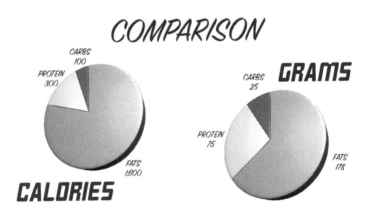

Upon first glance you might think, "Wow, my entire plate will be covered with fats." Because of the calories-to-gram conversion, it doesn't quite work that way, though. Many of my meals consist of a large salad topped with grilled chicken, a hard-boiled egg on the side, and guacamole somewhere on the plate. We'll discuss specific foods you can eat later in the book.

When you make the shift, something radical happens: "Your body changes from a sugar-burner to a fat-burner."[60] That is, you transition from a glucose-based metabolism to a fat-based metabolism.

Confused? No worries. In the next few chapters we'll discuss each of the three macros in more detail.

------

[60] *Keto Clarity,* p32.

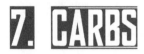
7. CARBS

MAIN IDEA: EVERYONE AGREES WE SHOULD EAT LESS SUGAR. THE PROBLEM IS THAT MOST PEOPLE DON'T UNDERSTAND WHAT ACTUALLY CONSTITUTES "SUGAR."

Everyone agrees our bodies function better with less sugar. *Everyone.* There's no disagreement about it. However, most people disagree as to what constitutes "sugar."

One doctor writes, "We have been told so many times that carbohydrates are good and fats are bad that we believe it to be a fact."[61] In other words, many of us believe two contradictory items about nutrition:

- Sugar is bad for you

- Carbohydrates are good for you

Most people are shocked to discover that all carbs act like sugar when they hit your bloodstream. In other words, the thought pattern should be changed to something more akin to the following:

- Sugar is bad for you

- Carbohydrates are sugar

---

61 *Dr. Colbert's Keto Zone Diet*, p4.

- Carbohydrates are, therefore, also bad

About twenty years ago I was at my wife's college apartment. School had just finished for the year, and everyone was moving out for the summer. At some point during the day I met the father of one of the gals who lived nearby. He was there, like everyone else, helping move his daughter back home.

Someone offered the two of us a drink- a soda.

"Sure, I'll take one," I said. This was back in my younger days when I could eat just about *anything* with minimal effect.

"What about you?" they asked the girl's father.

"No. I'll just take some water." Then- "I haven't had any sugar is over twenty years!"

I was shocked. I couldn't believe someone actually lived *without* eating sugar at all.

"What about birthdays and weddings and things like that? No cake?"

"None," he replied. "I don't eat *any* sugar."

"Why?"

"It's not good for you," he said. "I decided to completely cut it out of my diet decades ago."

I was perplexed. You see, not only did I find it hard to believe that someone could live without eating sugar- that they would just "give it up" forever- I also assumed that if you didn't eat sugar you'd be fit. Or, at least, you would look fit.

This guy didn't. He had the classic "dad bod." You know… skinny arms and legs, thick neck and double-chin, rounded-out-festively-plump belly. It's not "fat," but it's not fit- at all. It's something in "no man's land."

How in the world could *that* happen if you'd taken an oath to not eat sugar?

Turns out, the man had given up *some* sugar. He'd sincerely quit consuming the sugar he knew about. Candy bars. Cakes. Sodas. Pies. *Sweets*, in other words.

But he hadn't quit eating carbs. In fact, like most Americans, he consumed over half of his calories from carbs each day. That meant- get this- that **over half of his diet consisted of... yeah, sugar, *the very thing he'd sworn to avoid.***

In this chapter we'll discuss carbs in more detail. After making it this far into the book, you already know more than most people. Here, we'll take it one step further. Over the next few pages, we'll do the following:

- Identify four things you need to know about carbs

- Discuss what it means to "restrict" carbs and go "low-carb"

- Compare Atkins to Keto

Four things you need to know about carbs

Here are four things you need to know about carbs:

1. Carbs- *regardless of where you get them-* are sugar

2. Carbs- *regardless of where you get them-* act the same inside your body (except fiber)

3. Carbs aren't essential, that is, you don't have to eat them in order to provide your body with the nutrients it needs

4.   Carbs don't benefit *most* people

Let's walk through each of these.

First, carbs- *regardless of where you get them*- are sugar. I remember sitting at California Pizza Kitchen with the family the week after my wife started Keto.

"I'm getting a salad," she said. "Do you want to split the salad and split a soup, or do you want to split one and order something else, or do you want to go on your own?"

Up to that point, she and I had an unspoken plan anytime we ate at CPK. We always shared a salad *and* we also shared a pizza. By ordering two meals between us, we each got the best of both worlds. Her Keto experiment threw us off rhythm, because we couldn't order the pizza- even the gluten free option we usually ordered is full of carbs!

"We can still split the salad," I offered. "I'll add a soup or something."

"Ok," she replied. "I'm going to hold the tomatoes off my half of the salad. We can still get them, but we've got to get them on the side. And the croutons. Those need to go on the side, too. If you want them."

I understood the croutons. Those are just over-sized crunchy bread crumbs. Everybody knows bread is a carb, *but tomatoes*? Really?

"Why no tomatoes?" I asked.

"Carbs," she said. "I had no idea, but they're loaded with carbs."

As we talked about everything on that salad that contains carbs, it suddenly occurred to me that we bump into carbs all the time. In fact, when you start eating Keto you almost have to go out of your way to avoid them. (Within a week or so, you figure it out and it becomes super-easy. Or, you can take a look at the appendix of this book, get over the initial surprise of it all, and just move forward making wise decisions.)

What do we eat that contains carbs? The short answer: just about everything.[62]

For many people it starts with breakfast. A lot of people believe "I'm eating a healthy breakfast..." because they're *not* eating donuts. They're choosing *better*.

Look at breakfast this way, though:

- Orange juice is loaded with sugar- particularly when it's from concentrate

- Your coffee or tea doesn't have any carbs until you add honey and milk- then it's disproportionately loaded

- Oatmeal is a grain (a carb)

- French toast is bread, which is a carb (plus, we generally add loads of high fructose corn syrup- which is also a carb)

- Bananas have as many carbs as candy bars[63]

- Muffins and bagels = fancy bread = carb

- Cereal is a grain- and it's generally loaded with sugar as it floats in milk (which also contains sugar)

- Potatoes (including hash browns, breakfast potatoes, etc.) are also carbs

---

62 Because it's processed.

63 27g carbs per banana = 28g carbs per Snickers bar

Yes, first thing in the morning, most people *carb load,* thereby setting themselves up to be hungry all day while guaranteeing that their bodies will burn sugar instead of burning fat.

Here's why: your body interprets a bowl of M&Ms, a donut, a potato, a bagel, a banana, a cinnamon roll, or a loaf of bread as the same thing. **They all convert to glucose in your blood stream and, therefore, run the exact same macro.**

Each year the average American eats:

- 156 pounds of sugar

- 146 pounds of flour

That's 302 pounds of carbs right there, most of it starting first thing in the morning. That doesn't include fats and proteins- *that's just carbs![64]*

Your body treats all carbs the same

The second of four points I want to share with you about carbs is this: **carbs-** *regardless of where you get them-* **act the same inside your body**.

Think back to what Menotti said after he reanalyzed Ancel Keys study on the cause of heart disease. Keys said fat was to blame; Menotti said sugars were the culprit. He determined:

> *"Recognize that we are not just talking about table sugar or candy. The excess carbohydrates and starches we eat are eventually broken down to sugar. Carbs also come in the form*

---

[64] See *Eat Fat, Get Thin,* p15.

of fruits, bread, certain vegetables, potatoes, pasta, beverages, sauces, condiments, most dairy products, canned goods, desserts, yogurt, cereals, grains, wheat, corn, rice, oats, juices, and more."

I experienced the truth of Menotti's assertion first hand...

Last Fall, just before starting Keto, I hosted the semi-annual Advance workshop that I do with my friends Verick and Les each September and February. The schedule ran crazy-long on Saturday morning, then I needed to prep some things for the afternoon session, so I didn't have time to step out for lunch. No problem, I thought, I'll just run up to the Marriott Rewards hospitality room and grab something. Since we were hosting an event and had booked so many rooms, we had free access. They generally have finger foods like chicken fingers, so I could grab something quick and easy.

This was Saturday, though. Since most business people travel during the week, that's when they keep those hospitality rooms with complimentary goodies stocked. On the weekends, you fend for yourself from the assortment of fruits, yogurts and granola they keep on hand.

"That seems healthy enough," I told my friend Daniel.

He'd been helping me set some things up for the next session, so he lost his lunch break, too.

Over the next fifteen minutes I ate my "healthy" lunch. I grabbed a porcelain bowl and mixed in the following:

- Two small snack-sized cups of prepackaged yogurt

- Two tablespoons of pre-packaged honey

- About one 4 ounces of granola

- Two bananas that I sliced and put on top

MY "HEALTHY" LUNCH

	CALORIES	CARBS	OTHER NOTES
YOGURT	260	30	130 calories per container of Chobani yogurt, with 15g of carbs each- all of which is straight sugar.
HONEY	130	34	Honey has 65 calories per tablespoon, as well as 17g of carbs- all of which is sugar.
GRANOLA	100	19	I estimate I had 1/4 cup of granola. This contains 20g of carbs, but includes 1g of fiber- so 19g net carbs.
BANANAS	200	48	The bananas are about 100 calories each, contain 27g of carbs (minus 3g of fiber = 24g net carbs each)
TOTALS	690	131	*Notice that my snack lunch was basically MORE calories that a sit-down full lunch, and it was straight sugar! It included 6x the recommended daily dosage of carbs you'll eat on Keto.*

Although *none of that looks like sugar* (except the honey), *it's all sugar*. Within 15 minutes of eating I experienced a sugar rush. An hour later I physically crashed. And I felt bloated. My legs puffed up, my belt instantly felt tighter, and my arms felt heavy. I had no idea why, because- in my mind- I'd eaten a healthy snack lunch.

But the data doesn't lie. Look at the numbers on the chart. Almost 700 calories, including 131g of carbs (that is, *sugar*). As I wrote this manuscript, I pulled out my Lose It! app to track the numbers on a Snickers bar. Just to see. I learned that a regular sized candy bar has 250 calories, comprised of 32g of carbs.

Do the math. If I ate *three* Snickers bars for lunch I would have only consumed 750 calories, 96g of which would have been sugar. That is, I would have ingested a few more calories but 25% less sugar (a full candy bar's worth) by eating three Snickers bars than I ate by choosing a "healthy" lunch!

What would have been the healthier lunch option? Yeah, the macros show those options are almost identical.

Here's what my body did to those carbs:

- Some of is was used for immediate energy needs (though not much, because I had just been sitting around most of the morning)[65]

- More of it was converted to glycogen, topping off the reserves in my muscles, placing it nearby for my "on demand" needs later in the day (i.e., walking to the Alabama vs. Vanderbilt football game a few miles away)

- Most of it converted to fat stores on my body

Why? Because my body treats all carbs the same.[66] Yours does, too. They're the same macro, so they run the same command.

---

[65] Your body will only tolerate about 5-6g in bloodstream. That's about a teaspoon. Anything over that and you body strives to eliminate it.

[66] Exception: fiber. We'll talk about it in a few pages.

You don't actually need carbs

*I would have been better off that day had I not eaten the "healthy lunch,"
right?* In fact, I'd be better off if I never ate that lunch again. Ever.

Even though that concoction consists of things you likely eat *regularly*
(banana, yogurt, granola, honey), you'd be better off without it too,
right?

It's easy to make assessments like that and agree, "Yeah. That was a
waste of calories. I didn't need that. I'll skip it next time."

Here's the deal: you can actually skip that lunch every time. And you
can skip eating that for breakfast. And for snacks. **You see, your body
doesn't need carbs. That is (and this is our third of four
observations), carbs aren't essential.**

A lot people are surprised to learn that their body can make all the
glucose it needs. One author actually spelled it out plainly, observing
that "there's no such thing as a carbohydrate deficiency."[67]

I didn't believe it. After all, we've been told by the government to eat a
lot of carbs. So, I read a few books. Here's what I found:

> *"There is no such thing as an essential carbohydrate."*[68]

And,

> *"This is not true of fats, proteins, many vitamins, minerals,
> water, or fiber. If we don't get these nutrients from our diet, we
> develop [deficiencies]."*[69]

---

[67] *Keto Clarity*, p48.

[68] Nora Gedgaudas, quoted in *Keto Clarity*, p48.

[69] *The Ketogenic Diet*, p30.

Now, this flew in the face of everything I thought before studying Keto. Again, I'd heard the mantra over and over: eat more healthy carbs. Problem is, there aren't healthy ones. *They all run the glucose macro.*

What does the "glucose macro" do?

Again, **it uses some of the sugar for "quick energy."** Not as much as you might think, though. Your bloodstream will only hold about 5-6g of sugar (about a teaspoon) before your body seeks to *eliminate* it.

(No, you don't poop it out. That would be too convenient.)

The **second batch of glucose converts to glycogen stores**- your muscles are "topped off" with whatever deficit remains in the 1,600 calories or so which your muscles can hold.

Then, **the remainder of the glucose converts to instant fat.**

To this point in the book I haven't mentioned insulin. So, let's outline a few things insulin does, as it has an important function in your body.

- **First, insulin acts as the key that unlocks your cells and permits glucose to enter them.** In other words, Insulin is necessary for your body to use glucose as energy.

- **Second, insulin blocks the breakdown of fats.** When your body releases insulin it effectively sends sugar through the aforementioned process of quick energy, glycogen, and fat storage while at the same time blocking the use of fat for fuel. In effect, insulin tells your body, "Here, store fat instead of burning it for fuel."[70]

---

[70] "The main blocker of ketone production is insulin." See *Keto Clarity*, p78.

INSULIN = A KEY

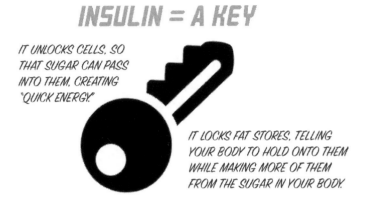

IT UNLOCKS CELLS, SO THAT SUGAR CAN PASS INTO THEM, CREATING "QUICK ENERGY."

IT LOCKS FAT STORES, TELLING YOUR BODY TO HOLD ONTO THEM WHILE MAKING MORE OF THEM FROM THE SUGAR IN YOUR BODY.

Back when I began running, I noticed that a lot of new long distance runners actually *gained* weight as they began running more.

In a word, here's why: *insulin*.

Runners are notoriously told to "carb load" before they run. The problem with carb loading, though, is that most of us don't perform at a level that requires us to carb load. If you're a world class athletes about to sprint for 400 meters, you may need to carb load. Your body *will* use the quick energy. For most of us, though, "carb loading" amounts to nothing more than managing our hunger, keeping us from getting a grumbly tummy during the middle of a long, slow run.

Here's what else carb loading does- it fills your body with insulin that quickly tells your body not to burn fat but to store it.
Furthermore, with time, you can become insulin resistant. That means your body has to produce more insulin to unlock the cells and eliminate the glucose from your blood stream. And, as a result, it means increased fat storage.

Do runners need carbs? No. Not really.

When runners "carb load" what they're really doing is eating something so they don't feel hungry while they're performing. Furthermore, the only reason they get hungry is because their body isn't trained to burn fat for fuel.

That leads us to another question: *What about the carbs you actually do need?* Remember, "surprising as it may be, we don't *need* to get our carbohydrates from our diet! it turns out that our bodies can make all the carbohydrates we need..."[71]

That's right, **your body can- and will- manufacture any carbs that you need**. I'll discuss, *gluconeogenesis*, the name for this process, in detail in chapter 9.

(For now, make a mental note that your body can only use a certain amount of protein. Any protein you ingest over the required amount is converted to glucose and is then treated just like a carb. So, although you don't want to overdo it on anything you're better off over-eating protein than over-eating carbs.)

Why do you need carbs, anyway?

The final observation I want to make about carbs is this: fourth, **carbs don't benefit most people**. Again, this flies directly in opposition to the common "wisdom" of our day, but it's true. Most people who eat carbs will gain weight- even if they're exercising regularly (like those runners).

In all my research I've found a few things that carbs are great at:

---

71 *The Ketogenic Diet,* p30 (emphasis added). Also, the name of this process is called gluconeogenesis. See the chapter on proteins for more info.

- Providing an extremely limited amount of quick energy (i.e., a "sugar rush")

- Communicating to your body to store fat

- Increasing your hunger (I'll explain this in the next chapter)

Do you want to accomplish any of those three? Look back at the list. **If a sugar rush, storing extra body fat, or getting hungry is a priority, then carbs might be your thing. If not, carbs aren't your friend.**

A few months ago, Mini and I made that monthly Costco grocery run again. It's not strange for Costco to have eight or ten sample stations spread throughout their big box warehouse. What is strange, though, is for the vendors to hand out samples of Ensure- a "healthy" shake used for adults who need to consume calories without consuming food. It's commonly used for people who don't have an appetite but need to insure they don't starve.

Though the Ensure website touts the drink as loaded with nutrition and boasts only 1g of sugar, here's what's actually in it: *carbs.* Lots of them.

I actually told the vendor, "This isn't healthy. This is actually *unhealthy.* I wouldn't want someone who is sick to drink this."

As I thought more about it I realized that if someone healthy drank enough of that shake it could actually make them feel sick. I know it would do that to me- I turned down the sample.

Then, as we browsed the shelves and looked at some of the generic brands, we learned the hard truth. Ensure was actually "healthier" (quotes used on purpose) than most of the other brands. The other brands didn't hide the sugar at all. Some of them had 30 and 40g of actual sugar in the form of sugar!

But it doesn't really matter whether they "hide" it or not, does it? All glucose works the same in your body.

My best guess as to why they include glucose in these "healthy" drinks is this:

> *"Nutritional guidance has long cautioned us to stay away from fat or risk getting fat, not to mention ending up with some terrible diseases; and worse, diet advice has given carbs a free pass."[72]*

And there are only three macros. **If you remove fat, you've removed the macro that provides the most taste.** Most foods, quite simply, don't taste good once your extract the fat. In order to make it palatable you've got to add something back in. The only option is to add protein or sugar. Which do you think tastes better?

Yeah, **the predisposition against eating fat actually pushes people from the most healthy option right towards the least healthy option.** The wisest option is to restrict your carb intake.

What does it mean to restrict carbs?

On Keto, your goal is to consume about 5% of your daily intake from carbs. Again, if you're eating 2,000 calories that amounts to 100 calories or less from carbs (25g).[73] For ketosis to occur, most people need to restrict their intake to the 20-30g net carbs.

---

72 *The Ketogenic Diet*, p41.

73 Carbs have 4 calories per gram, so 50g x 4 calories = 200 calories total.

That leads me to the next point. I've alluded to this quite a few times- and even discussed it in the previous chapter.

There are three types of carbs:

- Sugar

- Starch

- Fiber

The first two are the ones we want to stay away from. "In your body, whether it is a sugar, carb, or starch, it all registers as sugar in the end."[74] Fiber, though, is considered non-digestible. **Fiber passes through your system. As such, these don't count towards your overall carb count.**

WHEN COUNTING CARBS...

SUGAR

+ STARCH

- FIBER
_____

NET CARB COUNT

So, when counting your total carbs for the day, look only at the total number of carbs (sugars + starch) minus fiber. This is your net intake for the day.

_____

[74] *Dr. Colbert's Keto Zone Diet*, p86.

Going Keto will require an initial adjustment to your diet. The average man eats about 1,300 calories in carbs per day (the average woman eats about 950 calories)- *over half of their diet.*[75]

Yes, the average man over-eats in general. He consumes 2,700 calories- even though he only needs about 2,000. The average woman consumes about 1,850- more in line with what women need. Men tend to be the biggest over-eaters.

Notice, though, not only are most people over-eating, most people eat an abundance of carbs. Whereas only 5% of your dietary needs should come from carbs, most people actively eat *over ten times* that amount!

Here are four tips for restricting carbs:

- Eliminate breads, cereals, and grains of all kinds

- Avoid anything containing high fructose corn syrup

- Stop drinking your calories

- Take a close look at the fruits you eat

Let me explain.

First, eliminate breads, cereals, and grains of all kinds. This is a no-brainer. Go ahead and stop eating bread, pasta, cereal, oatmeal, bagels, muffins... anything made with wheat.

By the way, gluten still contains carbs, so going gluten free won't do the trick. You can literally purchase gluten free chips, gluten free tortillas, and gluten free bread. When running macros, your body doesn't care if

---

[75] This means the average man eats about 2,700 calories- even though he only needs about 2,000. The average woman consumes about 1,850- more in line with what women need. Men tend to be the biggest over-eaters.

it contains gluten or not. It will still run the macro for whatever kind of food it is.[76]

Second, avoid anything containing high fructose corn syrup. In fact, you should avoid *anything* that says "fructose" on it. It's usually accompanied by the prefix "high fructose" (as in high fructose corn syrup), but *all* fructose is unhealthy.

Fructose is "similar to glucose in shape and size," but there are significant differences. The most relevant for Keto is this: "fructose is used differently by the body."[77]

Most of the time when you read "fructose" on a label, it's referring to a syrup mixture that contains 55% fructose and 45% water & glucose mixed. Oddly enough, most table sugar is similar in content to fructose- it generally consists of 50% glucose and 50% fructose.

Here's why you need to stay away from it:

> "Like glucose, fructose is sent to the liver for metabolic processing after it passes the gut.

> "But while glucose heads off on a journey through the bloodstream, ultimately to be used up for energy by cells all over the body, fructose stays put in the liver, where it is converted to fat."[78]

Did you catch the path fructose takes in your body? Here's the comparison-

---

[76] Any sensitivity or allergy you have is an additional issue- added on top of this!

[77] See *The Ketogenic Diet*, p174.

[78] See *The Ketogenic Diet*, p174.

GLUCOSE vs. FRUCTOSE

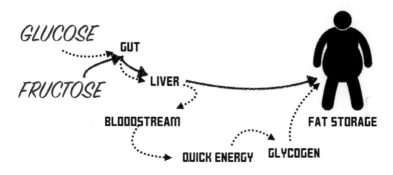

Whereas glucose runs through the blood stream, then is used for quick energy and fills glycogen reserves before moving to fat storage, **fructose moves straight to fat storage. It provides no energy to your body at all, as it bypasses the entire process of energy creation.**

There's no biological need for fructose. Be careful, though, because you'll find it in things labeled:

- Honey

- Agave

- Molasses

- Syrup

- Other sweeteners (read your food labels and the ingredients list)

All of these items above convert to glucose in your blood stream. And, yes, you may want to enjoy some of them in limited quantities while on

Keto. However, read the label and make sure you're ingesting the authentic ingredient and not some version of fructose masquerading as the real thing.

Now you know, too, why you can drink a few sodas over the weekend and instantly feel bigger. The truth is, well, you probably *are* a bit bigger.

That leads us to the third point: stop drinking your calories. It bears repeating: last year I heard that the average male would lose 25 pounds per year just by ceasing to drink calories- without any other dietary or exercise changes at all. The previous point, in part, explains why. Our drinks are loaded with junk calories that convert straight to body fat.

I know what you may be thinking. I'll just drink diet soft drinks. Turns out, they don't really work, either. Remember- carbs, protein, and fats are the three macros. Everything is one of these or it's a synthetic. (Synthetic is a fancy word that means "processed," that is, "created in a lab.") Generally, artificial sugar acts like sugar in your body and has even worse side effects!

Fourth, finally, evaluate the fruits you eat. I'm not saying you should stop eating fruits, but you need to do an honest assessment of what's in them. The truth is that the health benefits of some fruits have been drastically over-sold. At the same time, the harmful effects of fructose has been underplayed.

A lot of fruits contain naturally-occurring fructose. Most of them do, in fact. In the next few chapters we'll discuss why this matters to your overall health.

Why Atkins doesn't work long-term

Earlier in the book I referenced Dr. Atkins, the first modern physician to show the health benefits of a low-carb-high-fat diet back in the 70s. The main difference between Atkins and Keto is this: Atkins focused more on carb reduction and less on ketosis. That is, Keto focuses on eliminating carbs and ingesting more fats; Atkins focuses just on eliminating carbs. That's probably how you know the Atkins diet. It's common knowledge that "marketing for the Atkins diet has always focused more on carbohydrate restriction and less on ketosis."[79]

Notice the chart below. Though Atkins and Keto both focus on restricting carbs, there are some differences.

ATKINS / KETO COMPARISON

	CARBS	FATS	THE PLAN
ATKINS	Low	Doesn't specify high or low	Taper off, after a while, adding carbs back to your diet
KETO	Low	Always high fat	Continue with the low-carb-high-fat plan of eating, maintaining a state of ketosis

First, Atkins doesn't prescribe whether you should eat high-fat or low-fat in conjunction with the low-carbs. For this reason, a lot of

---

[79] Keto Clarity, p43.

Atkins dieters take more of a "Paleo" approach and fill their meal plan with protein. As we'll see in a few chapters, though, excess protein in the body actually converts to glucose and is treated just like a sugar.[80]

Second, Atkins encourages you to "taper" off the low-carb portion of the diet after you hit your desired weight. Gradually, you're supposed to add carbs back into your eating. Keto doesn't generally encourage this.

The progressive phases of Atkins systematically become less restrictive on carbs. The problem with adding carbs back becomes two-fold:

- Carbs convert to glucose, which becomes the first "go to" fuel for your body. In other words, it kicks you out of ketosis.

- Carbs also hijack your hunger hormones. Not only do they not satisfy you like fats do, they actually increase your desire to eat more.

Due to the "addictive" nature of carbs (who can eat just one chip, one bite of cake, etc.?), you continue eating more...

In reality, phases 3 and 4 of the Atkins diet (the place where you add more carbs) are where people can easily lose the discipline and give up- almost without realizing they are. Their taste buds adjust, they eat more and more glucose, their body kicks out of ketosis, and they stop doing the things that created the great weight-loss gains in the first place.

Make sense?

---

80 One authors writes, "Atkins guides dieters first through a ketogenic diet for rapid weight loss and then progresses to a less restrictive eating pattern that is considered low-carb compared to the average diet but which is no longer ketogenic above a certain threshold (about 50-60g of carbs per day)" (The Ketogenic Diet, p250).

That's a wrap

Let's go back to our two assumptions- that your health is dependent on eliminating toxins and shoring up deficiencies, and that when you do your body becomes self-healing.

Questions...

- In light of what you've just learned about carbs, are they a toxin or a nutrient?

- Are they helpful or are they harmful?

Yeah, that makes it easy to evaluate their place in our diet, doesn't it?

In the next chapter we'll tackle the issue of hunger. Carbs make you hungrier. And if you're hungry, your body will sabotage what you're working to accomplish, and you'll find it impossible to lose weight.

8. WHY YOU ATE BUT STILL FEEL HUNGRY

MAIN IDEA: FOR ANY DIET TO WORK YOU'VE GOT TO MANAGE YOUR HUNGER. IF YOU DON'T, YOUR BODY WILL WORK AGAINST YOU, SABOTAGING YOUR WEIGHT LOSS.

For any diet to work, you've got to be able to control your hunger. If not, you'll eventually give up. This is, in large part, why starvation diets don't work. In fact, starvation diets make you irritable, and you don't see results quick enough. Eventually, you give up, most often gaining back more weight than you originally lost.

The first time I lost all of my weight, I worked on simple calorie cuts. Thus, when my wife told me she was going Keto, that she was going to lose weight and listed all of the foods she was going to enjoy (particularly when she mentioned the word *fat*), I thought she was crazy.

As I was studying the Keto diet, I found a great quote that speaks to this: "Nutrition is far more complex than just counting calories."[81]

---

[81] *Bulletproof Diet*, p42.

Think about, though. **If dieting success was as simple as consuming less than you burn, a starvation diet *would* work.** It would work every time you tried it.

But they don't work, so we've got to dig deeper and determine what's really happening if we want to lose weight effectively.

Last Fall I started working-out at a gym outside of my home- at a new interval training gym known as F-45. I'd spent the previous few years working out via Beach Body DVDs, online streaming workout sets, and running. I was ready to make a change. When a friend from church mentioned he'd just opened a gym and that the first week was free, I decided to give it a shot.

I met some incredible people at the gym from all walks of life. I met athletes, soccer moms, stay-at-home-dads, female professionals, and people who were struggling to lose weight.

One day Hesston, the owner of the gym, had the "pod guy" visit the gym. The pod guy has a truck that carries a water tank that tells you your body fat composition when you jump in. It's supposed to be a far more accurate than body fat calibers- and is certainly more reliable than the height-weight charts you've seen which merely see people as two-dimensional entities.

One of the ladies jumped in the pod guy's machine one evening then returned to the gym the next day with some devastating news. "He said I'm obese."

I looked at her. She didn't *look* obese. I mean, she's in her late 50s, so she doesn't look like she's twenty. *But obese…? That was a bit of a stretch.*

"What did he tell you to do?" I asked.

"He said I need to cut back. I need to go to 1,200 calories a day."

"What? That's like half of what I eat," I replied. "How in the world can you...?"

A week later, she walked into the gym dejected.

Then- "I've been doing this for seven days," she said, "and I've only lost one pound. I'm miserable, I'm hungry all the time, and I'm not making any progress. None."

My first instinct was that she's clearly *cheating* on the diet. I mean, eat 1,200 calories and the math suggests that you're going to drop weight. *Quick.*

But, maybe not. Maybe the answer is not that simple. In fact, over the next few pages I'll argue that she wasn't cheating, and that the cards were actually stacked against her making any progress at all.

They give you free appetizers, because...

Like I mentioned before, I take my daughters on a "date night" the first Thursday of every month. It's a standing commitment we have- one that I hope runs all the way until the day they get married.

Every single month we decide we'll try something *new* for dinner, but every single month we go back to the Cheesecake Factory. Unless it's too cold or wet, we always dine on the outdoor patio. Oh, and *they always bring out lots of bread.*

Makes you wonder why they bring all those baskets of bread, doesn't it? After all, portions sizes of their entrees are colossal, and a huge part of their profit margin is built around the fact that we'll have enough room left in our bellies for cheesecake. Seems like with big portions and so much riding on the post-dinner purchase, they'd want to give us *less* food at the beginning of our meal for free instead of more food, right?

Well, here's the reality. "Wheat and related grains are potent appetite *stimulants*."[82] That's right. All the free bread actually makes you *hungrier*, almost guaranteeing that you'll spend more money and buy more cheesecake!

Ever been to a Mexican restaurant and turned down the free chips and salsa? Probably not.

Have they ever "cut you off" after a few baskets? No. The chips are grain-based, also guaranteeing that you'll not only not be able to eat just one chip but you'll also eat more burritos and tacos and enchiladas after you do.

Remember, bread is a carb. Chips are carbs. That means they're both sugar-based, which makes you hungry, hungry, hungry.

Why carbs make you hungrier

Sugar makes you hungry (remember, carbs = glucose = sugar) because of your body's appetite hormones and what it does to them. In other words, the issue is biological. It's a result of what your digestive system does when certain macros are introduced.

You have two main hunger hormones:

- Leptin- *decreases hunger*

---

82 William Davis, "Wheat and Hunger," http://www.wheatbellyblog.com/2015/08/what-makes-you-hungry. Emphasis mine.

- Ghrelin- *increases hunger*

Notably, each of these hormones are turned "off" and "on" by the foods we eat. That is, they don't control you. Rather, you control them.[83]

It's important to understand *how* to control them, because- as one doctor writes- "It is next to *impossible* to lose weight when your own appetite is sabotaging you."[84]

Let me talk you through these hormones, because it's easy to get confused as to how they work.

First, let's talk about leptin, the hormone that *decreases* hunger.

Leptin is produced in our body's fatty tissue. Because of this, obese people usually have *more* of it, which would lead you to think they might feel full most of the time. Things don't work that way, though. *If you have too much leptin you actually build resistance to it.*[85]

Leptin is present in foods that are high in fat, too, which is why you eat them and suddenly feel full. However, if your body is *already* carrying too much leptin, it requires more being introduced for your body to get the signal and then say, "Hey, I'm full. Stop eating, now."

In other words, it takes more leptin (and, hence, eating more food, thereby consuming more calories) to feel full. As you might imagine,

---

83 The signals for each can be changed by aging, obesity, and foods with additives.

84 *Dr. Colbert's Keto Zone Diet*, p130, emphasis added.

85 "Leptin is produced by fat cells, and your leptin levels are proportionate to your body fat levels. This means the fatter you are, the more leptin you have in your body" (*Bulletproof Diet*, p13).

that means that you eat more than you normally would have- all because your body can't process the proper signals.[86]

Second, let's discuss ghrelin, the hormone that *increases* hunger.

Ghrelin is a hormone your body naturally produces, as well, to let you know it's time to eat. If you've ever skipped a meal and then felt hunger urges a few hours later you've experienced the power of ghrelin.

In those moments of primal hunger, your body is pumping out ghrelin, effectively communicating, "Feed me!"

Get this, though. **Your body not only releases ghrelin when you haven't eaten, it also pumps out gherlin *as a response to carbs in your system!*** In other words, when you go to the restaurant and start munching on free bread and limitless bowls of chips, your body goes into over-drive, creating a *hungrier* sensation than you had when you first walked into the restaurant. That's why your will power vanishes once you start munching chips.

My best guess it that my friend at the gym did a bunch of calorie counting and determined that the best thing she could cut and still have enough food on her plate was fats. After all, whereas carbs only have 4 calories per grams, fats have 9. Logically, you can have over twice the amount of food if you're eating carbs, right?

Well, *not really.* Remember, fats are a more dense form a nutrient. That means they have more energy and more good fuel that your body can use. And, when you eat fats you actually feel full (in part, because of the leptin). Plus, when you devour a carb, your body releases the ghrelin, thereby *commanding* your body to continue eating.

---

[86] "Sensitizing you to leptin ensures that you only feel hungry when you actually need food" (*Bulletproof Diet*, p14).

By eating carbs, she took a "lesser" fuel source over a better one. And, in the process, she created an environment in which her body began begging her for more food. (I'm not saying she ate it, but I am saying that's why she was hungry.)

Notice how this works:

- Fat in your diet helps you control ghrelin, because leptin says, "Hey, we're full. No food needed."

- Carbs cause your body to release more ghrelin, saying, "We're about to starve- eat now!"

In other words...

- If you don't eat, your body releases ghrelin- and tells you that you're hungry

- If you eat carbs, your body releases ghrelin- and tells you that you're hungry

Either way, you feel hungry and your body *sabotages* your appetite.

And don't forget about insulin

Remember, whenever we eat glucose we've got to deal with insulin, too.

Now, to be clear, insulin isn't "bad." It's truly a powerful hormone which your body needs. Insulin works by binding to cells and allowing sugar to pass into them, thereby causing the cell to use that sugar for energy. In other words, your body requires insulin to put sugar to work.

But, if we ingest too much glucose, our insulin levels skyrocket. Whenever your body senses glucose in your system, insulin does the following:

- Converts the first batch of glucose to "quick energy."

- Fill up the glycogen stores in your muscles

Once the glycogen stores are full, your body does two things that will prevent you from losing weight.

- Converts the rest to fat (for future use)

- *Blocks* fat from burning (i.e., tells your body to use any available glucose, whether it's in your blood stream or the glycogen stored in your muscles)[87]

Remember, the carbs have just increased your ghrelin output, too- so you're generating *more hunger* while also creating more fat storage.

I know. You're wondering why this happens, why God created us this way.

Let's think about it logically. Go back to the hunter-gatherer days of our ancestors. When fruits were growing, it was important that they ate *and continued eating*. They needed fat stores on their bodies, because the winter days were coming when plants and produce wouldn't be as readily available. And, a lot of the animals they hunted would hibernate or prove more difficult to find and kill. They needed to burn some quick energy for their current use *and* store fat for future use.

(This explains, too, why they ate fruit. All that fructose, recall, converts straight to fat storage.)

_____

[87] "Carbs turn on the metabolic switch, causing a spike in the hormone insulin, and this leads to fat storage" (Mark Hyman, *Eat Fat, Get Thin*, p14).

In other words, some insulin is a good thing. Here's the issue with it, though. In the same way you can become leptin resistant (meaning it requires more of it to do its job of communicating that you're no longer hungry), you can also become insulin resistant. This means it requires *more* insulin to do the job of removing glucose (read: sugar) from your blood stream. So, when your body senses that glucose is present, it begins pumping insulin in order to convert the glucose to energy in your cells.

But- *and this is huge-* if you're insulin resistant it requires *more* insulin to the the job- meaning you actually release more.

Why is more insulin an issue?

Two reasons. First, insulin promotes the conversion of extra glucose to fat. Your body becomes more efficient at storing fat. Second, since insulin blocks your body from releasing fats as fuel, your body becomes more adept and hanging on to those fat stores.

Remember my friend at the gym? This is where she found herself- hungry (because of the gherkin), but still at the same weight (because of the fat storage issues created by insulin).

Why you can't eat like you did when you were younger

When I was in college, I could eat an entire pizza and not gain a pound. Now, it seems that if I eat two slices of pizza I can actually feel my "love handles" grow a bit. You've probably experienced something similar. You eat too much of something and feel bloated, you sense that your thighs have grown, or you feel that your waistline instantly expands.

As you age you naturally become more carb sensitive *and* insulin resistant. Here's what that means:

- **Carb sensitive** = less carbs create more issues for you, their effects are amplified in your body

- **Insulin resistant** = your body burns more in order to tell it what to do with the carbs, thereby instructing your body to store even more fat (i.e., it takes more insulin to remove the glucose from your blood stream- yet, all the while, the insulin is storing fat)

A lot of people decide to "work around" this sugar dilemma by using artificial sweeteners.

"If sugar is bad," they say, "I'll just eat something else."

Remember, though, the only "something else" that you can eat are fats and proteins. That's it. We've only got three macros.

That said, artificial sweeteners are *more bad news regarding your hunger hormones.* A University of Sydney study determined that artificial sweeteners are demonstrated to increase caloric intake by 30% or more![88]

Why? Because your body can't do anything with a synthetic. **Your body only metabolizes natural products.** So, your brain has to recalibrate in order to figure out what you're feeding it.

When you ingest fake "sugar" here's what occurs:

- Your blood sugar levels *don't* rise like normal.

---

[88] *Dr. Colbert's Keto Zone Diet*, p135.

- The brain senses that you're eating, but it doesn't receive the total message. It never senses satiety. Therefore, your body continues requesting more food for the body.

The result? You get hungrier- just as you do when ghrelin is released.

Have you ever grabbed a diet soda and wondered why you suddenly craved more food? Or another drink? *That's an example of this.* Diet sodas generally trigger the appetite and cause sugar cravings.

Furthermore, not only can the body not "do anything" with the fake sugar, it's a toxin. Your body can't break it down. And, remember (as we discussed earlier in the book) one of the biggest issues with health is shoring up your deficiencies while eliminating toxins.

Dr. Colbert writes,

> "High fructose corn syrup, MSG, and artificial sweeteners are additives that do not add anything of value to your body. They will sabotage your weight loss, create food cravings, imbalance your appetite hormones, cause insulin spikes, and program you for obesity."[89]

That's a pretty good reason to stay away from artificial stuff.

The final analysis

Now, let's put it all together.

- Leptin (found in body fat and in fat foods) creates a feeling satiety. You feel satisfied, full.

---

[89] *Dr. Colbert's Keto Zone Diet*, pp137-138.

- Ghrelin (found in your body and generated by carbs) produces feelings of ravenous hunger. It produces the "eat now or we'll die" kind of feeling.

- Insulin is required by your body to allow glucose to pass through your cell's walls and convert to energy.

But, too much of any of this creates a domino effect.

- Too much leptin builds a resistance, thereby requiring more fat to reach satiety.

- Too much ghrelin causes you to feel even hungrier.

- Too much insulin causes your body to continue storing glucose as body fat while- at the same time- preventing body fat from being converted to usable energy.

The result of any of these three scenarios is that you feel hungry- even if you're eating. You see, it's possible to consume a lot of calories and still feel like you've just missed a meal.

9. PROTEIN

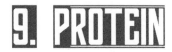

---

*MAIN IDEA: PROTEIN IS ONE OF THE MACROS THAT ARE
ESSENTIAL TO YOUR BODY'S NEEDS (THE OTHER BEING FAT). TOO
MUCH PROTEIN, HOWEVER, MITIGATES AGAINST YOUR HEALTH.*

I've got another friend who owns a different kind of gym- not the cross-fit, interval training type I mentioned earlier. He owns the kind of gym where guys lift heavy weights and drink protein powder like it's a thirst quencher. (Some of the guys there even eat it by the scoop rather than mixing it with water or milk!)

One day he told me, "Those guys are nuts. They used to only drink it after the work out. But the biggest trend now is the pre-workout. They actually load up before they do anything."

"Instead of afterwards?" I asked.

"No," he answered. "They dose up on protein powder before the workout and after the workout. Both!"

I'd been studying Keto and the unique effects each of the three macros have on our bodies, so I asked him, "Do they know what protein actually does? Or have they just heard that they need more of it, so they've just blindly followed along?"

"I'm not sure," he replied. Then- "What exactly does it do?"

Now, it wasn't surprising to me that he didn't know. He's a business man. An entrepreneur. He happens to own a gym because it produces a recurring stream of revenue and it's a much healthier and livelier option than other business which he could potentially own. Aside from the economic impact his location generates for the neighborhood, he offers an incredible service to the community. People look better and feel stronger because of what he does. I don't have any qualms, in other words, about the fact that he's a businessman who owns a gym.

I gave him the standard line I'd read in a book:

> *"Protein is used in the body for building and repair of muscle tissue, and for various enzymatic functions. Normally, your body spares protein for those purposes and doesn't use much for energy."*[90]

Then I explained to him, "Most people don't know that last part- the energy part. They assume that protein is the *creme de la creme* when it comes to energy for building muscle. So, they overdue it. They assume that more is better. It's not."

"Really?" he said, "Does it matter?"

"Turns out, it does," I explained. "You see, your body will only use the protein it needs. You can't store extra protein. So, your body has to do something with it. **The only means you have of storing *anything* in your body is to store it as body fat.** So, your body converts extra protein into glucose and then, after topping off your glycogen stores, packs on more body fat."

"Why don't most lifters know this?" he asked.

"Because most lifters aren't nutritionists. *Most lifters just lift.* They haven't made the correlation that food is fuel. And that your body does

---

[90] *The Ketogenic Diet*, p27. Emphasis mine.

specific things with each kind of fuel. This explains, though, why some guys who lift a lot can never get *ripped*. Or *cut*. It's why they lift and their muscles just get puffier instead of more defined. Too much protein. It converts to fat and fills in all the gaps of any muscular definition they would otherwise have."

But... your body needs protein

Whereas as carbohydrates are not essential (i.e., you don't have to supply your body with them by eating them), *protein is essential.* In fact, **of the five macros we're mentioned in this book, only 2 are necessary to eat- protein and fats.** That means you must ingest some protein in order to meet your body's needs.

Here's a great overview of protein and what your body does with it:

"...the body avoids using proteins for energy because they have so many other important functions. Muscles, organs, bones, and skin are made of protein. The enzymes that catalyze the reactions in our body are 90% protein. Antibodies, the important immune system responders that fight infection are protein. Some hormones, like insulin, are also proteins [some hormones are fats]. Some proteins, like hemoglobin and albumin, carry things around in our blood...

"Because proteins are essential to so many body systems, the body prioritizes using proteins to replenish the machinery rather than breaking them down for energy. So long as we eat

enough calories to meet our needs, proteins will be 'spared' for these other functions."[91]

If you don't consume protein, your body will face several potentially severe consequences.

Notice the following points from the quote above:

- Protein comprises the building blocks of your muscles, organs, bones, and skin. In other words, *you are protein.*
- Protein is responsible for many of your hormones, enzymes, and antibodies.
- Protein isn't actually a significant source of energy, because your body uses it for those other important functions.

Yeah, we need protein.

The issue with protein is this: **because it's necessary, people overdue it. They tend to overestimate how much they need.** Or, they never do the math. They just assume that "more" is always better.

How much do you need? Turns out, *not that much.* A little goes a long way.

Don Colbert, a noted doctor, suggests you consume 1g per kg of body weight (1kg = 2.2 pounds).[92] This gives us the following recommendations at the following body weights:

- 210 pounds = 95g
- 195 pounds = 88.64g

91 *The Ketogenic Diet*, p75. Emphasis added.

92 *Keto Zone Diet*, p118.

- 180 pounds = 80g

- 165 pounds = 75g

- 150 pounds = 68.18g

The Keto diet suggests you consume 15% of your daily calories from protein. On a 2,000 calorie diet that amounts to about 300 calories / 75g. Notice the numbers above and look at the chart below. This 15% provides enough protein for the average 165 pound person. If you weigh more or less, you just make the adjustments necessary.

TARGET RATIOS, ASSUMING 2,000 CALORIES/DAY

	% OF DIET	CALORIES	GRAMS
FATS	80%	1,600	178
PROTEIN	15%	300	75
CARBS	5%	100	25

By the way, your body can recycle protein- as much as 300g each day. If you consistently eat your daily allotment of 15% (approximately 300g) you'll be in great shape.

The question then becomes, *"Now that I know how much protein I need, where do I get it? And do I have to eat a lot of meat in order to do so?"*

Let's answer both of those questions. There are many sources for protein- and they're not all meat products. In fact, you can ingest plenty of protein without eating meat at all.[93]

For instance, seafood and poultry are great sources of protein. But so are eggs (7g each) and cheeses.[94] In fact, here is a list of low-carb-high-protein-foods:

- Almonds

- Avocado (also high in fat, making it a great Keto food)

- Black beans

- Cheese (try Mozzarella, for instance, as well as plant-base cheeses)

- Chia seeds

- Deli meat (read the label first)

- Edamame

- Eggs[95]

- Fish

- Greek yogurt (check the brand- some are loaded with carbs)

---

[93] For instance, Rich Roll is an ultra athlete who happens to be a vegetarian. Go to http://www.richroll.com for more on how he supplies himself with plenty of protein with a strictly plant-based diet.

[94] Search https://www.womenshealthmag.com/food/high-protein-low-carbohydrate-foods/slide/20 or https://www.eatthis.com/high-protein-low-carb-snacks/, both accessed 04-25-2018.

[95] Eggs are a great staple for Keto, because they are also high in fat. And, they have every essential amino acid. See *Dr. Colbert's Keto Zone Diet*, p116.

- Hemp seeds

- Jerky

- Lentils

- Peanut butter (just don't get one that's loaded with sugar)

- Pistachios

- Quinoa

- Tuna salad

Remember, you don't need as much protein as many people initially think. If you're going to drink a protein shake, make sure that you don't blend it into milk (high in sugar) or add a stack of bananas to it (straight carbs). As well, make sure the protein shake doesn't throw you over your actual dietary needs.

Note: there are a few potential pitfalls you can fall into when looking for sources of protein. Namely, the additives:

- Condiments placed on protein usually adds a lot of calories in the form of carbs (in other words, the chicken is great- but the sauce slathered on it is horrible)

- Some meats, like BBQ, contains a lot of added sugar when prepared (again, due to the sauce)

- Frying and flouring any kind of chicken or beef coats the protein with a layer of carbs

- Processed meats generally have added sugars and synthetic fillers which your body treats like a carb

A great side effect of eating protein is that your body actually has a feedback loop that turns your cravings "off" when you eat it. Here's how it happens:

> "When your small intestines detect protein in the food you've eaten, it helps leptin stimulate satiety."[96]

This assumes, of course, that your hunger hormones are working properly (i.e., that you're avoiding carbs, so that they're not hijacking them into a feeding frenzy).

Now, I've warned you about eating too much protein. So let me explain- in more detail- why you need to make sure you don't overdue it.

Gluconeogenesis: what happens when you overload on protein

Yes, there is a potential pitfall of protein: *eating too much of it.* I began the chapter talking about how a group of muscle heads at a local gym kept overloading on protein powders. Here's the issue:

> "Our bodies can't store excess protein, it has to be used. When we consume too much protein, our bodies convert much of it into glucose through a process called gluconeogenesis. This can increase blood glucose levels and keep you from achieving ketosis."[97]

When you ingest protein two things happen.

---

96 *Bulletproof Diet,* p28.

97 Maria Emmerich, quoted in *Keto Clarity,* p76.

First, your body first captures what it needs to maintain bone density, muscle mass, etc. Again, protein is *essential*, meaning that we must eat it in order to keep these important body functions working properly.

Second, your body stores excess protein, but it stores it the only way it knows how to store unused macros- as fat. Your body can't actually do anything with any extra protein you consume, so it gets rid of it through a process of *gluconeogenesis*.

I know. I just gave you that big word. Again, when we break apart the word *gluconeogenesis* we get an accurate mental picture of what the word means:

- Gluco = glucose

- *Neo* = new

- *Genesis* = create

That is, **your body creates new glucose from the protein overage.** It does this, for the most part, in the liver. Then, it releases the new glucose into your blood stream just like it does when you eat carbs.

(WHAT DOES YOUR BODY DO WITH EXTRA PROTEIN?)

GLUCONEOGENESIS
GLUCO-   NEO-   GENESIS
GLUCOSE   NEWLY   CREATED

You shouldn't be *scared* of *gluconeogenesis*. This process allows your body to to make its own carbs from protein, ensuring that you don't have to eat carbs.

What do we do, then?

Eat your protein. But keep it in the allotments mentioned in the chapter- 1g per kg of body weight.

Protein is one of the macros essential to your body's needs (the other being fat). Too much protein, however, mitigates against your health.

10. FOOD PYRAMID SCHEME

MAIN IDEA: THE FOOD PYRAMID CREATED BY THE GOVERNMENT IS ONE BIG SCHEME. BASED MORE ON ECONOMICS AND COMMODITIES THAN ACTUAL HEALTH AND NUTRITION NEEDS. IF YOU EAT BASED ON THEIR PYRAMID YOU'LL GAIN WEIGHT AND, IN ALL LIKELIHOOD, STUMBLE INTO SEVERAL HEALTH ISSUES.

I remember sitting through Ms. Patterson's first grade class and learning about "The Four Food Groups."[98] If you're anywhere near my age, you probably remember them, too. Back in the day when elementary schools had art classes, music programs, and school nurses the food groups were branded into our little brains.

I remember all four:

1. Milk & dairy

2. Meat

3. Bread & cereal

---

[98] The four food groups were called "The Basic Four," and were promoted by the government from 1956 until 1992.

4. Fruits & vegetables

THE 4 FOOD GROUPS

* REFLECTED THE HIGH-CARB, ANTI-FAT BIAS

* SEPARATED FOODS BASED ON WHAT THEY LOOKED + TASTED LIKE RATHER THAN WHAT THEY DO IN THE BODY (EX: MANY FRUITS & GRAINS ACT THE SAME, B/C OF THE CARB COUNT)

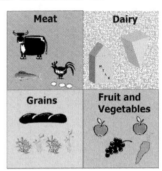

Homeroom teachers and school nurses instructed us to eat a specific number of servings from each group every day. If we did, we were promised we would be healthy.

"You'll grow big and strong," they said.

Now, I don't think they were tricking us at all. Our teachers were just as uninformed as everyone else. They just spouted the "party line" we'd all been given.

By now you know the truth, though. The food groups don't accurately reflect *anything* about how our bodies handle the food or what our bodies even need. You know, for instance, that-

- Your body treats breads and some fruits the same, like sugar.

- Your body treats some milk like a fat and other milk like a sugar.[99]

- Your body treats some cheese like a protein, other cheese like a fat, and other cheese like a carb.

- Your body treats some vegetables like a carb and others like a protein.

- Your body responds to meats based on how you cooked them and whether you floured them or just grilled them (and if you loaded them with condiments or not).

In other words, the four food groups reflect how we categorize items in the supermarket and how we place them on our plates. Really, though, they don't speak much to nutrition.

The scheme

In 1992, the year I graduated high school, the government shifted its focus from the four food groups to the "Food Pyramid." Though the USDA revised the pyramid to a different emphasis in 2010 ("choose your plate"), then released a *different* set of guidelines in 2015 (which are good through 2020), the recommendations remained basically the same as you might expect having read this far through the book:

- Stay away from fat

- Eat more carbs

---

[99] Despite the ad campaign that dairy farmers- coupled with the government- ran in the mid-to-late-eighties, milk does not "do the body good." The way we manufacture it, anyway. We load it with sugar!

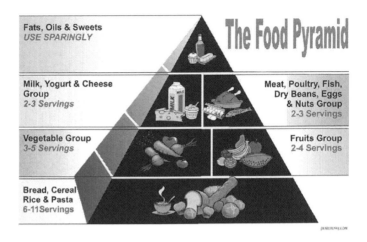

In fact, the 2015-2020 Dietary Guidelines suggest 45-65% of your calories come from carbs.[100] Even if you stay on the low side of their recommendations, you'll eat almost ten times the amount of carbs recommended on Keto. **By now, you know that if you follow those guidelines on the pyramid above, *you'll get fat.*[101]**

Let's start at the bottom of the pyramid, work our way up, and making a few observations along the way.

First, the government recommends you load up on breads, cereal, rice, and pasta. Since we've already invested 20 pages together talking about carbs in general (chapter 7), followed by another 10 discussing why you get hungry when you eat them (chapter 8), we'll move to our next observation about the pyramid.

---

100 Source: http://health.gov/dietaryguidelines/2015/guidelines

101 "The average person, if eating the low-fat, high-carb diet as instructed by every medical, food, nutrition, and government agency, will most likely continued to gain more and more weight" (Dr. Colbert's Keto Zone Diet, p30).

DON'T EAT THIS

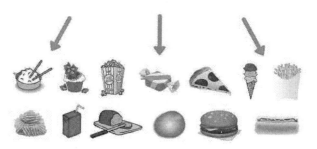

Second, "fruits and vegetables" both require a more complex guideline than just "eat ____ amount." Here's why: *we don't evaluate foods based on what we call them, we evaluate them based on the macro and what they do.*

Fruits and vegetables are *not* the same, regardless of where you place them on the pyramid.

- Some vegetables are high in fiber (i.e., spinach, broccoli). They don't count towards your carb count, and they actually empower your body to digest food more readily.

- Most fruits are high in sugar (bananas, apples). They'll *explode* your carb allowance for the day.

One researcher reminds us, "Fruits actually have more in common with candy than they do with vegetables."[102]

---

[102] *Bulletproof Diet*, p34.

He adds, "The health benefits of fruits are over-stated while the health risks of fructose are completely ignored."[103]

The fructose that fills most fruits causes them to increase your appetite while packing weight on *immediately*. This makes fruit a better option for desert than for a "healthy side."

By the way, dried fruit and fruit smoothies are often worse for you than fruit picked straight from the tree. When the fruit is "dried-out" or blended into drinkable form, the fruit is compacted and more dense. That means you have all the sugar in an easier- and less satiating- form.

And you generally have far more of it:

- I can eat an entire bag of dried fruit in one sitting. That might be the equivalent of a dozen or more peaches. It's a catatonic load of sugar!

- I can drink a smoothie created from 5-6 apples, 5-6 bananas, and a cup of strawberries- *even though I would never be able to eat that much fruit in a single day*.

See how that works?

Let's move on up the pyramid...

Third, milk, yogurt, and cheese can come in different forms, too. A few chapters ago I told you my yogurt story. And I've detailed how milk interacts with your body differently based on the amount of fat or sugar that's in it. This means that this category is not a "one size fits all" option.

Fourth, fats- the cornerstone of Keto- are listed with sweets. Remember, though, sugar is a *carb*. Ancel Keys' lead researcher,

---

[103] *Bulletproof Diet*, p35.

Menotti, characterized carbs as sweets. Fats are, well… *fats*. Most oils are fats (though not all). We'll discuss fats in chapter 11.

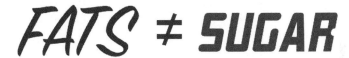

FATS ≠ SUGAR

(CARBS = SUGAR & SWEETS)

Fifth, finally, the pyramid recommends *far too much food for one person* to eat in a day. Take a look at the pyramid and count the number of servings recommended:

- If you eat the maximum amount of servings of each item you'll ingest 26 servings of *something* per day.

- If you eat the minimum, you'll still eat 15 servings.

Quite simply, either extreme is way too much. Regardless of what kind of food you eat, if you eat that much, you'll gain weight.

Again, **the government makes recommendations here based on what the food looks like instead of coaching us nutritionally** based on what the food does in our bodies, based on the macros the foods run.

Why would they...?

All of this leads us to a few questions, candid ones like-

- *Why does the government ignore the last fifty years of health history?*

- *How does the government not see what everyone else plainly sees?*

A few months ago I found myself scrolling through Netflix on a lazy Sunday afternoon. Eventually I came across a strange-named documentary that caught my attention, *Fat Head.*[104] In the film, Tom Naughton argues that the government has fed us, in his own words, a "load of bologna" in telling us that foods with fat are bad for us.

The main reason they do this- *again, in his words-* is economic. He says it's hard for the government to on one hand push commodities like corn while on the other hand telling us how bad corn-based products (like high fructose corn syrup) are for us.

In other words, to summarize his argument, *"Follow the money."*

I love how Wikipedia says it outright, too:

> *"The guides have been updated over time, to adopt new scientific findings and new public health marketing techniques. Over time they have described from 4 to 11 food groups."*[105]

Again, we've been recommended foods based not on what the foods do for us but what the money we spend on food can do for the economy.

---

[104] http://www.fathead-movie.com

[105] https://en.wikipedia.org/wiki/History_of_USDA_nutrition_guides, accessed 04-25-2018, emphasis added.

The USDA actually revises their guidelines based on economic decisions before releasing their findings. And, yes, they negotiate the terms behind closed doors, before they give those recommendations to me to you.

Remember the food pyramid released back in the nineties? The pyramid we saw isn't the first pyramid they wanted to release. Here's the scoop:

> *"The first chart suggested to the USDA by nutritional experts in 1992 featured fruits and vegetables as the biggest group, not breads.* **This chart was overturned at the hand of special interests** *in the grain, meat, and dairy industries, all of which are heavily subsidized by the USDA."*[106]

As you might imagine, it's hard to do real science when money is over-involved.

An article in the *British Medical Journal* states that the U.S. nutrition advice is suspect, that it doesn't stand up to scientific standards:

> *"The scientific committee advising the U.S. government has not used standard methods for most of its analyses and instead relies heavily on systematic reviews from professional bodies such as the American Heart Association and the American College of Cardiology, which are heavily supported by food and drug companies."*[107]

---

[106] https://en.wikipedia.org/wiki/History_of_USDA_nutrition_guides, accessed 04-25-2018, emphasis added.

[107] See Nina Teicholz, "The scientific report guiding the US dietary guidelines: is it scientific?," in the *British Medical Journal*. Emphasis added.

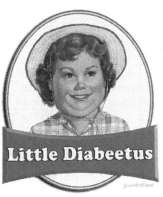

SUGAR-
IN ANY FORM!

- *IT DOESN'T HAVE TO COME IN THE WRAPPING OF A SNACK CAKE- IT CAN COME PACKAGED AS A FRUIT, AS A BREAD, AS ANY CARB...*

- *YOUR BODY RESPONDS TO IT THE SAME.*

Little Diabeetus

Furthermore, an article in *Mayo Clinic Proceedings* actually stated that the food pyramid is "incompatible with human survival."[108]

How is the food pyramid inconsistent with health? Well, I pulled the following graphic off the Internet...

Initially, the first time I saw it, I thought, "Yeah. Snack cakes and candy bars are bad for you! And sodas! We eat and drink too much junk!"

Remember, though, the most important issue is now what the food is *called* or *where we place it in the supermarket* or *where we chart it on the pyramid.* **The most important issue is the macro- the macro denotes what "command" the food follows when it enters your body.** Regardless of whether you package a carb in the form of bread, macaroni, bananas, cereal, sports drinks, or Little Debbie snack cakes, the result is the same. *They're all the same macro.*

---

108 http://www.mayoclinicproceedings.org/article/S0025-6196(15)00797-1/fulltext, accessed 4-25-2018.

The crazy carb cycle

Since Ancel Keys first labelled fat as "bad" several decades ago, the food industry and the medical community have aligned their interests. Here's what we've seen on a mass-scale, what you'll see (or may have already even seen) on your own:

- **First, health issues emerge.** Someone has an issue for which they want healing (it could be the desire to lose weight, or any other thing).

- **Second, they follow the medical community + food industry's recommendation of removing the fat from their diet.** Because fat provides taste (and nutrition), something has to replace it. Since there are only two macros left, you can add protein or carbs. Carbs taste better- because they're glucose (read: *sugar*).

- **Third, more issues surface as a result of the carbo-centric diet.** The person seeking to eat their way out of health issue finds themselves eating the one thing that shuts down your immune system, causes you to gain more weight, and instigates an entirely new set of additional health issues.[109] Oh, they end up eating a diet consisting almost entirely of processed foods, too. The result is that they get sicker or heavier.

- **Fourth, they "double down" on the diet.** Ironically, instead of looking for the root causes of the health problems, they go "all in" with the high carb option recommended by the government. As one doctor writes, "Rather than going to the root of the problem, which is the

---

[109] Processed = not natural / less nutritious AND has the additives

food we are eating, our habit is to address the symptoms."[110] Yes, this is same government from whom they adamantly *won't* take budgeting advice, productivity hacks, or parenting tips- because we all know better.

Thus, the cycle just continues, eventually spiraling out of control until it reaches epidemic proportions.

CRAZY CARB CYCLE

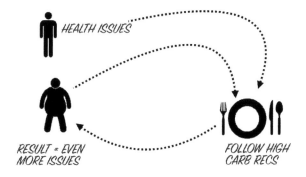

HEALTH ISSUES

RESULT = EVEN
MORE ISSUES

FOLLOW HIGH
CARB RECS

At some point you've got to step out of that cycle, right? Or, to say it another way, you've got to jump off the pyramid!

I know what you're probably thinking: *there are people who actually recommend carbs.* Trainers encourage clients to eat them, and doctors suggest people eat them.

In actuality, most trainers are experts in muscles and movement- *not nutrition.* Would the manager at the local gym really push excessive use of protein powder if he knew what it did in the body? Would that trainer

---

110 *Dr. Colbert's Keto Zone Diet*, p32.

insist on carb-loading if she knew that carb-loading just abates hunger pains and pushes more food to fat stores in your body- all while spiking your blood sugar?

Probably not...

Furthermore, most doctors are *specialists*. That means they have an extremely high level of expertise in a specific area- *but not all areas.*

I wouldn't take advice from a gynecologist about my prostate. Nor would you take advice from a neurologist about your foot. In the same way, if you want great nutrition advice, seek the guidance of an expert... someone skilled in nutrition.

And seek the help of someone who looks at things from a preventative-health standpoint rather than a reactive-only point-of-view. And someone who enjoys natural options instead of synthetic ones.

Remember where we began the book? Yeah, if you remove the toxins and bring in the nutrients, your body will heal itself.

And that leads us to the final macro, the one that brings the largest array of nutritional benefit to your body. It's time to talk about fats...

11. FATS

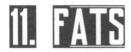

MAIN IDEA: WHEN YOU EAT FATS(S), YOUR BODY FIRST BURNS THE FATS YOU EAT. THEN, AS IT NEEDS MORE FUEL IT MOVES TO THE FAT STORES ALREADY IN YOUR BODY.

So here we are... we're at the third and final macro we'll study, *fats.* As I mentioned earlier in the book, when my wife told me she was "going Keto," I winced. Grimaced. I thought, *Surely that can't be right? Eating a bunch of fat? Surely she knows that won't work...*

Turns out, she was right. *I was wrong.*

To go Keto myself, I had to "get over" my initial fear of fat. You will, too.

In fact, **if you don't "get over" the fat-issue, you won't succeed at Keto.** Here's why: **Fats are the cornerstone of Keto.** Most of your calories come from fat- not protein. And definitely not carbs.

What's a cornerstone? Well, back in the era of huge cathedrals and in the early days of building skyscrapers, builders first measured their foundation. After pouring it, they set a key stone in place. Usually over-sized and obvious, this *cornerstone* provided the reference point for erecting the remaining structure.

That's how fat works for the Keto diet. **Everything is built around the fat(s) macro.** It's the reference point, the building block, for everything else.

When you fuel your body with fats instead of carbs, your hunger hormones and brain communicate to your body, "Hey, finish up the remaining glucose and glycogen storage that we've got on hand, and then let's start burning fat."

And, "**Let's burn this fat we're eating, first. When we need *more* calories, let's burn up the fat already stored here on the body.** It has 9 calories a gram- over twice the amount of the carbs we were burning anyway, so it's a rich, dense source of nutrition."

In response, your body starts burning fat *and* it releases *ketones* as a byproduct of burning that fat.[111] Those ketones are used for energy, primarily by the brain- which prefers to run on these fat-based products rather than glucose.[112] **When your body burns fat for fuel and releases these *ketones*, you're considered to be in a state of *ketosis*.** This is where the name Keto originates. All that said, if you don't eat enough fat, you'll thwart ketosis.

How much fat do you need? **80% of your calories should come from fat, if possible.**

Now, this is exactly *the opposite* of the 2015 Dietary Guidelines of America, which suggest that only 20% of your caloric intake come from fat. **Remember, though, the only three macros you can consume for nutritional purposes are fats, proteins, and carbs.** If you eliminate- or strictly limit- fats, you'll by default make it up with one of

---

111 We mentioned earlier that ketones are also considered a macro.

112 Keep reading the main text, but here's a spoiler alert. The reason Keto works great for neurological issues- like ADD, ADHD, Alzheimer's, etc.- is because your suddenly *not* feeding your brain sugar.

TARGET RATIOS, ASSUMING 2,000 CALORIES/DAY

	% OF DIET	CALORIES	GRAMS
FATS	80%	1,600	178
PROTEIN	15%	300	75
CARBS	5%	100	25

the other two. The carbs will *always* convert to sugar; any protein your body can't use for it's already-designed purposes will transform to sugar as well. In the end, *if you follow their guidelines, you'll gain weight.*

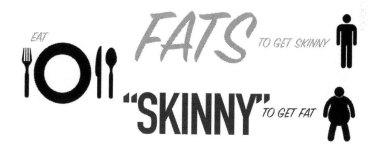

Remember the lady at Starbucks, the one who ordered the skinny latte? She'd bought into the notion that the way to get thin is to eat "skinny." She stood certain that if she ate fat she'd balloon up.

Going Keto sounds like the opposite of what most people think, doesn't it?

A lot of people think that fat in foods converts to body fat. When my wife told me her plans to eat a high-fat diet I was certain that's what would happen to her. Even though they have the same name, body fat and fat in foods are two different items altogether. A Harvard study noted: "The notion that food fat equals body fat isn't completely true, and the advice has been misguided."[113] Eating fat doesn't make you fat anymore than eating blueberries makes you blue.

Again, when both carbs and fats are both present in your body, your body will burn the carbs (glucose) first *every single time*. In some sense, this is your body's natural response to keep your blood sugar from going beyond the 5-6g range. The first overage replenishes the glycogen stores in your muscles; any additional overage converts to body fat. **To get thin, you've got to eat fat.**

Your body is comfortable with fats

Turns out, your body is actually *extremely* comfortable with fats- with the kind you eat *and* the kind stored in your body. Think logically with me. Your body goes into overdrive to eliminate glucose and convert it to a "safer" form, right?[114] But what does it do with fat? Yeah, it hangs onto it- unless you tell your body to use it by shifting into fat-burning mode.

Fat in foods:

- Satisfies (you're not hungry)

---

113 Referenced in *The Ketogenic Diet*, p20.

114 This is because sugar is a toxin!

- Nourishes (we'll discuss six benefits of Keto *beyond weight loss* in chapter 14)

- Provides better *total health* results than the other macros (see below)

Furthermore, since we've *already* decided to cut the carbs *almost completely out* and reduce proteins to what our bodies actually need, we're left with only three options of the macros we learned about just a few pages ago (see chapter 6):

- Fats

- Alchohol

- Ketones

Ketones are generated as the body breaks down fat. So, you must ingest fats to make ketones.[115] The only remaining macro is alcohol. Obviously, you can't live off *that*- even if King Solomon did write that "wine makes the heart merry."[116] This points to fat as our best option.

Of course, this doesn't mean that fat is a "consolation prize." Much to the contrary, it's actually what your body prefers!

In chapter 7 we learned that there are *no essential carbs*. You can reduce your carb intake to 0g and you'll be fine. (In fact, you won't just be fine, you'll likely watch your health prosper!)

---

[115] My advice about ketone supplements = don't. The reason you measure ketones is to evaluate whether or not your body is in ketosis, as ketones are the byproduct of your body doing the work of breaking down fat for fuel. If you ingest ketones in supplement form, you won't get an accurate assessment of where you are. The best option is to just eat enough fats and allow nature to run its course.

[116] See Ecclesiastes 10:19. Also, David says the same thing in Psalm 104:15.

Two of the macros *are* essential, however. That means you must ingest them in order to have them in your system.

- **Protein is essential.** In chapter 9 I mentioned that you must eat protein. It is essential, meaning that (aside from what your body recycles) if you don't eat it you don't get it.

- **Fats are essential.** We call the most important ones that are "essential fatty acids." There are two of these: Omega-3 and Omega-6. Generally, people get enough Omega-6 through their diet. Omega-3, though, often requires supplementation.

Notice this: "Fat is a building block of healthy cells and hormones and is needed for fertility, temperature regulation, and shock absorption. Some vitamins- A, E, D, and K- are fat soluble, meaning that they need fat in order to be absorbed in the body."[117] **Your body won't function properly without fat.**

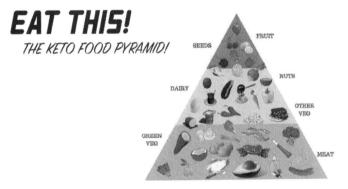

EAT THIS!
THE KETO FOOD PYRAMID!

SEEDS
FRUIT
DAIRY
NUTS
OTHER VEG
GREEN VEG
MEAT

SOURCE • WWW.LOWCARBALPHA.COM/KETO-DIET-FOOD-PYRAMID/

---

[117] *Bulletproof Diet*, p31.

(I placed an overview of the supplements I use in appendix C, including fish oil supplement. In my opinion, those are the best.)

Not all fats are created equal

One of the arguments people waged against the Atkins diet went something like, "Wait. You're telling me that you can't eat corn on the cob but you can eat a hot dog without the bun? Or you shouldn't eat bananas, but you can eat as much salami or bacon as you want?!"

No. Not exactly. All fats aren't created equal.

In the same way that NASCAR fuel isn't the same as the unleaded gas you pump at the quick-mart down the street, an organic hot dog isn't the same as a grass fed steak which isn't the same as a McDonald's Quarter Pounder. The quality of your food actually matters. It amazes me how many people will purchase the best tennis shoes for their feet or designer clothes for their back yet then skimp on the calories that fuel the body. Quality matters. Better food is better for you.

As well, the *kind* matters. In the same way there are different kinds of carbs there are different types of fats:

- Saturated fats
- Unsaturated fats
- Monounsaturated fats
- Polyunsaturated fats
- Trans fats

Let's differentiate them just a bit:

Saturated fats. Most animal fats are saturated. When people speak against fats, they're generally arguing against these. Wiki reports that "the effect of saturated fat on cardiovascular disease is controversial." In other words, this is the particular fat- *out of all five of them*- that carb-enthusiasts target.

Throughout this book, I've argued the other side, that this fat is good for you, too. As Dr. Mercola writes,

> *"A misguided fallacy that persists to this day is the belief that saturated fat will increase your risk of heart disease and heart attacks. This is simply another myth that has been harming your health for the last 30 or 40 years.*
>
> *"The truth is, **saturated fats** from animal and vegetable sources provide **a concentrated source of energy** in your diet, and they provide the **building blocks for cell membranes and a variety of hormones and hormone-like substances.**"*[118]

Saturated fats and trans fats are the only two fats listed on the updated FDA food labels. We'll talk more about why in a moment.

(Oh, and don't get tripped-up as to why these fats are named what they are. It has more to do with their atoms, their bonds, and their chemical structure. It's chemistry, in other words. And though that's important, we can hit the high points and move on.)

Unsaturated fats. In general, plants and fish fats are unsaturated. If you have an aversion to saturated fats, you can still reach your fat intake by eating less saturated fats and more unsaturated fats. If you don't have an aversion to them, this gives you yet another set of food choices.

---

[118] https://articles.mercola.com/sites/articles/archive/2009/09/22/7-reasons-to-eat-more-saturated-fat.aspx, accessed 4-29-2018, emphasis added.

Whatever you do, though, *don't eliminate fat from your diet.* Fat is "actually required for numerous functions in your body related to growth and reproduction. Stripping all fat from your diet has negative health consequences."[119]

On Keto, it's not as important that you eat *saturated* or *unsaturated.* Rather, it's important that you eat *fat.* The kind is up to you.

Monounsaturated fats. *Mono* means "one." Monounsaturated fats contain one double bond in their fatty acid chain. "Monounsaturated fats (MUFAs) are good fats. Liquid at room temperature, they turn solid when they are chilled. Common sources of MUFAs are olive oil, avocados and nuts."[120]

Studies show that MUFAs help you feel less hungry, resulting in decreased irritability. As such, these fats make great on-the-go snacks.

Polyunsaturated fats. Whereas monounsaturated fats contain one double bond, polyunsatured fats (PUFAs) contain more than one double bond in their fatty acid chain. Omega-3 fatty acids are PUFAs, as are sardines, tuna, and wild salmon.

Trans fats. This breed of fats are processed by machines in industrial complexes. As such, *they're not healthy at all.* Crisco, shortenings, and chips & snacks you purchase from vending machines are often loaded with these toxins. The American Medical Association supports *eliminating* these completely.

Here's what's interesting. On the food labels (required by law for manufacturers of prepackaged food to publish), the FDA doesn't

---

[119] See http://healthyeating.sfgate.com/saturated-vs-unsaturated-fats-lipids-8611.html, accessed 4-29-2018.

[120] https://bodyecology.com/articles/6_benefits_monosaturated_fats.php, accessed 4-27-2018.

mandate that all kinds of fats be included on the label. In the same way that they only require 2 of the 3 carbs, they only require 2 of the 5 fats.

FATS & NUTRITION LABELS

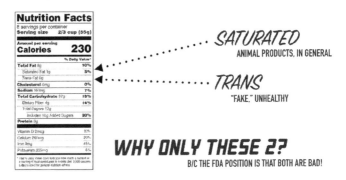

The FDA *seems* to argue that trans fats and saturated fats are both equally bad for you. In fact, most articles that I've reviewed which speak against high fat diets don't argue against all fats, they argue against these two. Furthermore, they go head-to-head with the saturated fats more often than the trans fats.

Personally, I've found saturated fats to be a pleasant staple in my diet. They provide satiety, they taste great, and they help me eat "more normal" in a variety of situations- all while staying on my nutrition plan.

If you don't want to eat saturated fats, though, there area few things for you to consider.

First, there are plenty of fats you can eat that *aren't* saturated fats. Notice that you can eat fish, plants, and nuts to acquire the fats you need. (See also appendix A for an actual list of Keto-friendly foods.)

Remember that, in general...

- Saturated = animal products (i.e., red meat, eggs, chicken, dairy)

- Unsaturated = fish, plants

- Monounsaturated = olive oil, avocado, nuts

- Polyunsaturated = small fish- like sardines, tuna, salmon

- Trans = fake, processed!

In other words, you can still reach your fat requirement without eating red meat if you choose to do so.

Second, removing saturated fats from your diet may not actually make a huge difference- unless you already eat a numerous amount of them. Let me explain...

Someone warned me about eating too much steak. They said it could be bad. Now, they had no proof of it or any reason why it could be bad; *they'd just heard it somewhere.*

I don't eat steak every day, though. I only eat it once every few weeks.

I don't eat burgers every week, either.

To make a health change that makes a difference, there has to be a *meaningful change* in your common, everyday activities. If you only do something randomly and change *that*, it won't make a big difference. In this instance, eliminating steak or burgers- or both- from my diet wouldn't make a dent in my nutrition.

Why? Because I don't eat either one enough to make a meaningful difference. I already limit these items.

Now, the American Heart Association (AHA) suggests you limit the following items in your diet:[121]

- Fatty beef

- Lamb

- Pork

- Poultry with skin

- Beef fat (tallow)

- Cream

- Butter

- Cheese

- Other dairy products made from whole or reduced-fat (2 percent) milk.

Notice this list. It's kinda like my steak, isn't it- other than the butter? These are foods I eat *randomly*, for the most part.

Well, I drink some milk with my coffee. But I generally use heavy cream or whole milk. (The skimmer versions the AHA actually recommends are *loaded* with sugar.)

Here's what all this means: most people's health *will not* make a dramatic uptick by removing saturated fats from their diet. Most of us don't eat enough bacon, steak, or eggs to pin them as a health issue, anyway.

On the other hand, there are several things that most people do eat every day. Yes. Every. Single. Day.

---

121 http://www.heart.org/HEARTORG/HealthyLiving/FatsAndOils/Fats101/Saturated-Fats_UCM_301110_Article.jsp#.WuNrhy_Mz-Y, accessed 4-27-2018.

- Sodas and/or sugar "sports" drinks[122]

- Dairy like milk and ice cream

- Grain in the form of bread, muffins, cereal, oatmeal, crackers

- Starches in the form of rice, pasta, potatoes

- Bananas and apples

The American Medical Association (AMA) suggests a similar eating pattern to the American Heart Association (AHA) guidelines which we just referenced. The AMA says:

"To get the nutrients you need, eat a dietary pattern that emphasizes:

- *fruits, vegetables,*

- *whole grains,*

- *low-fat dairy products,*

- *poultry, fish and nuts,*

- *while limiting red meat and sugary foods and beverages.*

Choose lean meats and poultry without skin and prepare them without added saturated and trans fat.[123]

You should replace foods high in saturated fats with foods high in monounsaturated and/or polyunsaturated fats. This means

---

[122] Go read the label on Gatorade or Powerade. Both are the nutritional equivalent of slurping down a candy bar.

[123] Notice these two kinds of fats. They're arguing- wrongly- that saturated fats and trans fats are the same.

eating foods made with liquid vegetable oil but not tropical oils. It also means eating fish and nuts. You also might try to replace some of the meat you eat with beans or legumes.

In general, you can't go wrong eating more fruits, vegetables, whole grains and fewer calories."[124]

Again, look at their list and do some critical thinking. Fruits and vegetables aren't the same- so let's eat the vegetables and evaluate the fruits we eat. Let's eliminate the whole grains, so that we can avoid the carbs. Let's choose milk with fat in it instead of milk which has been modified to contain more sugar. Let's eat the fish, poultry, and nuts they suggest. And the beans. And, sure, let's not eat red meat for every meal. Also, let's definitely avoid the sugary sodas.

By the way, you should- as much as possible- *eliminate* processed foods from your diet. If it's processed, that means it's been created in a lab. The World Health Organization (WHO) recently classified processed meats as a carcinogen.[125] A carcinogen is a substance or agent that's known to cause cancer.

The importance of metabolism

Once people get over their aversion to eating "fat" in their diet (and understand that fat doesn't make you fat), there's another issue most people have to address. Namely, the calorie count.

---

[124] http://www.heart.org/HEARTORG/HealthyLiving/FatsAndOils/Fats101/Saturated-Fats_UCM_301110_Article.jsp#.WuNrhy_Mz-Y, accessed 4-27-2018.

[125] Stacy Simon, "World Health Organization Says Processed Meat Causes Cancer," *American Cancer Society*, October 26, 2015.

CALORIE COMPARISON OF THE THREE MACROS

	CALORIES / GRAM
CARBS	4
PROTEIN	4
FATS	9

Earlier in the book I provided you with a chart similar to the one above. It clearly shows that fats hold more than *twice* the number of calories that carbs and proteins have.

Remember, though, **calories aren't just numbers; they represent units of usable energy. And, the way your body handles those calories is determined by their macro.**

We typically think of metabolism as "how fast we burn food." And, since most diets are based on caloric restriction, we generally assume that less calories is always better. This leads many people to avoid fats like the plague- due to that larger number.

But metabolism is broader than just burning food. Metabolism includes "all of the processes that occur within a living organism to maintain life."[126] Sure, it includes how fast you burn food for fuel, but it's so much more. Metabolism includes basic functions like:

- Breathing

- Cellular division

- Circulation + blood flow

- Core body temperature

- DNA replication

- Heart beat

- Muscle repair

- Nerve signals

Basal metabolism is the term used to denote what's required for these basics. The average adult needs about 1,200-1,400 calories for basal metabolism- just to stay alive. Everything else fuels your daily activities.

Again, metabolism *includes* the energy we use- and that energy comes from *both* the nutrients we consume *and* the process of converting stored energy (read: body fat) into fuel.[127]

Here's the bigger issue as it relates to nutrition- it works like your car:

- **Good fuel = *good performance***

- **Bad fuel = *bad performance***

---

[126] Quoted in *The Ketogenic Diet*, p72.

[127] "You're not metabolically healthy if you cannot access your fat reserves for energy" (See https://www.paleohacks.com/fat/eating-fat-vs-burning-stored-body-fat-20890, accessed 4-28-2018).

Food isn't just a resource to satisfy hunger pains; food is fuel. You don't have a dashboard with a fuel gauge to tell you when you're empty. Rather, you have hunger pains. They communicate to your body that it's time to fuel up. **Fat provides a "higher octane" fuel and, as we've demonstrated throughout this book, it performs better in your body.**

Furthermore: **if you cut calories below that 1,200-1,400 range (i.e, a starvation diet), your body *lowers* its basal rate and hang on to calories. In effect, you'll need to expend more energy in order to burn more fuel to avoid gaining weight or to lose weight.** This is what causes many calorie-cutting diets to plateau after a few weeks. Your body begins to cling to whatever calories it can rather than releasing them.

Keto has the significant advantage over other diets in that:

- Your body will be running on higher octane fuel

- Your basal metabolism remains higher, burning calories instead of "hanging on" to them

- The fuel gets better results

Is a faster metabolism always better?

That said, let me make a statement which might defy conventional weight loss wisdom. Here it is: don't worry so much about your metabolism, because *a faster metabolism isn't necessarily better.*

Our ancestors- even people living just 100 years ago- would never have thought, "Hmm, I'd really love a *faster* metabolism. I want my food to run through me quicker, I want to burn calories more efficiently. I want to be able to eat more food to meet my daily needs."

No, they'd want their nutrition to *last*. They wanted a slower metabolism. They'd view a faster metabolism as almost *wasteful*.

Think about your vehicle. We began our Keto discussion by comparing our bodies to different kinds of engines and different types of fuel. Do you want a car that burns through gas faster or one that burns through gas *slower* and *better*?

That's what I thought. You probably want better gas mileage, so you want the fuel to last longer.

One more question. Your family budget. Do you want your money to spend money more efficiently, that is quicker? Or do you want to spend it more effectively, that is, to "stretch" the dollars more?

Again, the answer is that you want the resource to last for more time, you want more mileage, you want a better deal...

It's odd, then, that we flip the discussion when we start talking about food and our metabolism. You see, if your body burns through nutrition faster, it means you're accomplishing less with each calorie.

In the end, you'll burn through body fat while on Keto. But it won't simply be an issue of a "faster metabolism" that makes it happen. Again, a faster burn isn't necessarily better when it comes to gas, money, or even (as our ancestors knew) food. The issue is whether you want to burn fat or burn sugar. Burning fat is always better. And, regardless of how fast or how slow you're burning it, if you're using the correct fuel, you'll lose weight. And you'll do so without going hungry, without growing tired, and without getting irritable. That's the promise of Keto. And it begins by getting comfortable with a high fat diet.

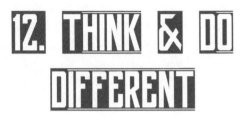

12. THINK & DO DIFFERENT

MAIN IDEA: TO GET DIFFERENT RESULTS THAN YOU'VE GOTTEN BEFORE, YOU'LL NEED TO ADJUST A FEW OF THE THINGS YOU'VE HISTORICALLY DONE. THINK + DO DIFFERENT.

A few years ago, right after I dropped my 40-plus pounds, I bumped into a friend at a Saturday workshop my wife and I were teaching. He was in the middle of a 30-plus pound drop himself- *all with a unique twist.*

"I'm taking this as far as I can *without* exercise," Chris said.

"None?" I asked him.

"*None.* I want to see what my body will do without it. You got a minute? I'll tell you about it."

In the same way I was certain that my wife's high-fat diet would make her highly fat, I was positive that this guy's non-exercising weight loss plan would backfire. But, having known him for a while, I thought I'd hear him out. After all, *would could it hurt to just listen?*

"I think too many people put the emphasis on exercising to lose the weight," he said. Then- "They end up over-thinking what they achieved, over-celebrating by rewarding themselves with snack treats, and they put the calories right back in their body. We're in a busy season of life right now. I don't have time for the next six months or so to possibly fit anything else into the schedule. I don't want to wait until it's more convenient to start losing the weight I need to drop, so I'm going to jump in and do it with diet. I'll add exercise later."

This made all the sense in the world to me. I remembered running 6-8 miles at a stretch when I was 50 pounds heavier. That was good for a 600 calorie burn. Later in the day, though, I'd chug one of my venti-sized white chocolate mochas from Starbucks (with added caramel syrup), rationalizing I'd "earned it" with my run. In doing so, I placed 720 calories of straight sugar back in my body. I would have been nutritionally in a better position if I'd skipped both the run and the drink. The combo put me in a 120 calorie deficit- and it was straight glucose. No wonder I gained weight consistently!

No, I wasn't about to stop exercising because Chris told me he was going to lose his weight while not exercising. I'm one of the guys who actually enjoys fitness. I look forward to getting stronger. I enjoy donning the headphones and heading out the back door of my house for a long-run, uncertain as to the exact route I might take in the morning- only knowing I will return 90 minutes or so later.

But here was a guy that wasn't anti-exercise. Nor was he waiting to start getting in shape until he could exercise. And his stance made me really wonder, "Can you do this without having to burn so many calories in the gym, on the treadmill, or with the Beach Body workout playing on the DVD player?"

In this chapter, I want to discuss that further. I and want to talk about a few other concepts I think we might need to adjust in our minds. You see, to get different results than you've gotten before, you'll need to adjust a few of the things you've historically done.

Here are four things I'd like us to consider over the next few pages:

1. First, eat for weight loss; exercise for strength & mobility

2. Second, eat based on macros- not food "groups" or "pyramids"

3. Third, stop counting calories

4. Fourth, treat carbs as potential toxins instead of quick energy

First, eat for weight loss; exercise for strength & mobility

Until recently, every weight loss routine I tried consistently mostly of "just go exercise more than you've been doing before" (which, in most cases, had been no movement at all). My theory was that, in no time at all, I'd drop the weight and see noticeable results.

I think this is actually the prevalent theory in our culture. Follow me here. At the beginning of the year, what does everyone do? Yeah, they join a gym. They don't necessarily change their plan of nutrition. Rather, they opt for a few laps on the treadmill or a few heaves of a weighted dumbbell.

A few years ago (yes, in January), I placed the P90X DVD in the small television in our office. I pulled myself out of bed at 5:30am that morning, so that I could start- and finish- before any of the small kids got up and needed help grabbing breakfast or getting dressed.

It was miserable.

Somewhere in the first few minutes of the routine, Tony Horton said something like, "You've got to eat right. No Krispy Kremes. If you don't eat right, you'll work out and you'll never look fit."

Eat right? What? This was news to me.

Somehow, in my mind I had separated eating right *from* working out *from* fitness. I thought you needed the second but not the first.

As I reflect back, my experience proves otherwise-

- *Remember how I actually stopped exercising for a season and still lost 15 pounds on Keto- even after I'd already lost 40?* I talked about it in chapter 5.

- *Remember those muscles heads at my friend's gym, the guys who power-up on the protein powder that effectively converts to glucose and puts a thin later of fat between their muscles?* I discussed it in chapter 9.

- *Remember my past experience with struggling for years to get fit, yet not being able to lose weight regardless of how hard I tried?* It's all in the intro to the book.

While researching to write this book, I came across the following quote. Pay attention, because if runs counter to just about everything you've heard regarding weight loss.

> *"One of the greatest misconceptions when it comes to weight loss is that burning calories is relevant to losing pounds and slimming down. That's because your diet is much more important than exercise when it comes to weight loss."*[128]

You see it, don't you? Yeah, Dave Asprey- the author of Bulletproof Die*t*, the book in which I found the quote- argues against the method I'd used

---

[128]

as my sole means of striving to lose weight before, simply by burning calories.

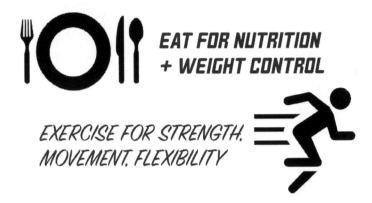

EAT FOR NUTRITION + WEIGHT CONTROL

EXERCISE FOR STRENGTH, MOVEMENT, FLEXIBILITY

Think about it logically, though, by way of two questions.

First question- *It is easier to burn calories in the gym or to just not eat those calories in the first place?* Most of us over-estimate how many calories we burn and underestimate how many we consume. It's easier to just not eat them, right?

- *A quick-tempo hour-long run through my neighborhood of rolling hills burns about 600 calories.* That's less than my favorite Starbucks drink- the one I don't order anymore. And it's about half of a slice of cheesecake I can split with my girls on date night.

- *A 45-minute high-intensity interval workout at F45 (a local gym I frequent) eats up about 400 calories.* That's a large bowl of ice cream, some cereal and milk, or a burger.

- A 25-minute set of Shaun T's "T-25" workout burns about 250 calories. That's a candy bar, two bananas, or a soda.

No, you'll never outrun a bad diet. I can't. You can't. No one can.

Second question- *How many of the calories that you burn do you actually have control over?* Originally, I would have thought, "All of them. I can control all of by choosing to be active rather than sedentary."

Now, you're not going to hear any argument from me that you should stop exercising. Or that you shouldn't start. But, think about this number: **50% of the calories you burn are based on things you can't control.**[129] That is, your metabolism is impacted by things like-

- Room temperature

- Sleep

- Altitude

- Breathing

And, yes, your brain uses about 500 calories per day just by being in the "on" position. That makes your noggin the single biggest calorie burner for most people.

Now, let's go back to our vehicle analogy. Earlier in the book we admitted that an automobile's gas mileage has as much to do with outside factors that it does the amount of fuel in the tank. In fact, we decided that the promise of "X miles per gallon" is simply a pipe dream, some far-fetched marketing ploy the manufacturers like to slap on the door to make us feel better about the purchase.

Look at the items on the graphic below- all factors that radically influence the rate at which your car burns fuel (i.e., gas mileage).

---

[129] *Bulletproof Diet*, p33.

- Some factors depend on the driver. Things like the speed he drives. How well he's kept the car tuned up.

- Some factors depend on things clearly outside of the driver's control. The weather. The road. How much traffic is present. City miles and highway miles.

- A few items depend on the car itself. The age of the car, the make and model, and the amount of cargo... these are factors related to the car itself.

MILEAGE MAY VARY

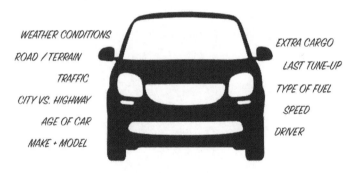

WEATHER CONDITIONS
ROAD / TERRAIN
TRAFFIC
CITY VS. HIGHWAY
AGE OF CAR
MAKE + MODEL

EXTRA CARGO
LAST TUNE-UP
TYPE OF FUEL
SPEED
DRIVER

The same is true for your body. There are numerous factors determining your rate of burn. Dave Asprey writes, "80 to 90 percent of what your body looks like depends on what you eat."[130] He adds, "Your diet is more important than exercise in determine the shape of your body and how you feel."[131]

---

130 *Bulletproof Diet*, p114.

131 *Bulletproof Diet*, p122.

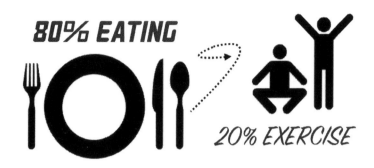

Again, I *am not* arguing against exercise. I am arguing against exercise as the sole means of losing weight, and I am arguing that you have more control over what you eat than you do how fast your body burns calories.

By the way, some people wonder if they can get lean without exercising. Turns out, I did.

After taking a few months off from the gym (in large part, to test the Keto diet), I made a work trip to Mobile. Instead of crashing at a hotel, I decided to stay with some friends and save the money.

One of my hosts, my friend Johnny (an amazingly fit guy who trains people professionally) looked at me and said, "Man, you've gotten ripped. What have you been doing to work out?"

I told him the truth, "Eating right. I haven't done anything physical since the first week of February- three months ago."

Again, I'm not arguing against exercise. I love physical activity. But, we need to determine the best "place" for exercise in our health plan. Here's how I now see it:

- **Eat for nutrition + weight control.** That is, manage your weight by watching what you eat.

- **Exercise for strength, movement, and flexibility.** That is, find a workout routine that challenges you and makes your heart, your muscles, and your lungs stronger.

Second, eat based on macros- not food "groups" or "pyramids"

This discussion about the primacy of nutrition over exercise leads us to the next thing we often get "backwards." This one is super-important, particularly since we've just acknowledged that you've got to use diet to reach your fitness goals- *even if* you're employing physical fitness as part of your overall health regimen.

A few years ago I watched the movie *Fight Club*.[132] Brad Pitt plays the part of a traveling soap salesman who serves as Edward Norton's alter ego, starts the namesake club of the film, and makes pithy statements throughout the story. Here's one of my favorites:

"Breakfast is just a myth put out by the cereal people."

Think about it. Long and hard. Especially in light of what you've read in this book.

Why do you eat breakfast?

Is it because you're actually hungry, or is it because somewhere you heard- *without any evidence to back it-* that breakfast is "the most

---

[132] https://www.imdb.com/title/tt0137523/

important meal of the day" and that if you don't eat breakfast your metabolism will slow down?

My guess is that it's the *second*. You received the myth as truth.

That said, don't just consider *why* we eat breakfast, think about *what we eat* for breakfast. Yes, carbs. We munch on things like bagels, muffins, toast, cereal... and, yes, orange juice. In other words, we carb-load first thing in the morning, virtually *insuring* that we'll crash mid-morning (right?!), that our hunger hormones won't work properly throughout the day.

(By the way, have you ever gotten a mid-afternoon slump- somewhere around 3:00pm? That's about the time you *should* carb crash from lunch.)

When we step back and look at food as fuel, a few new parameters emerge:

First, start eating whenever you *are* hungry and don't eat when you *are not*.

Sounds like a no-brainer, doesn't it? Problem is... well... we've been conditioned to eat at specific times, particularly in the West where there's an abundance of food.

- We've had it drilled in our heads that we must eat breakfast or our metabolism will go wonky.

- Around noon, we automatically start looking for something to eat- even if we're not hungry.

- About 5:30pm, same thing... we look for something to eat!

If my car has a full tank of gas, I don't pull into the gas station and "fill 'er up." Even if it's early in the morning. Or mid-afternoon. Or evening. Even if I'm on the way home from the gym which is when I generally gas up. That's irrelevant unless I need gas.

And food should be irrelevant unless you're hungry, right?

Here are two sure-fire ways to evaluate whether or not your body is actually in ketosis (read: burning fat for fuel) is if you can do the following two things:

- Wake up without eating breakfast, without feeling hungry until late in the morning.

- Exercise at high intensity without having to immediately eat afterwards.

Here's what these two observations reveal...

Your body signals it's "empty" by signaling your brain via hunger pains whenever it doesn't sense a readily available fuel source. If you've conditioned your body to crave sugar- particularly at short intervals throughout the day- you'll find yourself hungry immediately upon waking up. You'll need a soda, cereal, or even coffee.

Let me rewind and restate that final one, coffee. If you can take the coffee black, you might still be in ketosis. But, if you discover that your body really craves the milk and sugar, well... your body is commanding you to ingest carbs, simply using the coffee as the delivery mechanism.

Here's why this "test" works for exercise. Most people burn glucose whenever they go to the gym. They use whatever "quick energy" (read: blood sugar) is floating through their veins, followed by the glycogen that's stored in their muscles. After 30 minutes of that, most people feel depleted. As such, their body- fearing it will run out of fuel- begins craving a "top off."

When your body readily burns fat for fuel, it knows no such craving. Nor does it feel empty. It knows that there's a fuel source on standby- one that it can tap anytime it needs to. As such, you don't feel hungry for several hours into your morning, and you don't feel zapped as soon as you complete an intense round of exercise.

Makes complete sense, doesn't it?

Second, eat based on food categories rather than macros. A few pages ago we noted that the FDA and USDA categorized foods based on what they look like and where they go on your plate rather than what they do in your body. Hence, they lumped fruits and vegetables together. And they dropped candy in the category with fats rather than placing it with bread and cereal.

It's best to evaluate your fuel based on what it does in your body rather than how it looks like or what name you choose to call. When you do, you'll suddenly free yourself to eat better and make healthier decisions.

Suddenly, you'll notice things like:

- Eggs are a great option for supper- even if they are "breakfast."

- The left-over steak from last night's dinner… it's a good breakfast, if you're actually hungry for breakfast. If not, just eat it whenever you get hungry.

- Apples- *full of carbs*- make a great dessert instead of a "healthy side." After all, they have more in common with cheesecake than asparagus.

Again, the way to "think & do different" is to eat when you're hungry, and eat based on the macros instead of the name of the food.

This leads us right into a third thing we can do differently…

Third, stop counting calories

When you eat like I've just described, you'll discover that you can stop counting calories. There's no need to do it.

Besides, calorie counting simply frustrates most people. We've already learned that all calories aren't created equal, so looking at the caloric value only gives you partial truth.

That said, let me give you fair warning: **even on Keto you shouldn't eat more fuel than you burn.** If you do, you can still gain weight. Here's what happens on Keto:

- *Step 1*, your body first burns the fat in the food you're eating.

- *Step 2*, if you don't eat enough calories to fuel your daily needs, your body then turns to the fat that's already stored throughout your body.

Those points are important. If you eat more than what you actually need, your body remains in Step 1. You never get to Step 2, in other words, and you actually store the extra fat.

Now, I know what you're thinking: *How do I keep from falling into this trap? Do I need to count calories?*

The answer... is no. You just need to not eat unless your hungry.

A few years ago I had a co-worker who struggled to lose weight. He worked out five days a week, and he ate nothing but salads. It seemed like he should have been losing weight, because he did everything right:

- No carbs

- No sugary drinks or desserts

- No cheat days

Yet, not only did he fail to lose weight, *he actually began packing on a few pounds!*

Here's what I learned, as I look back at the time we spent together- me gaining weight on breaded buffalo chicken fingers and him gaining weight on salad. Quite simply, if your body requires 2,000 calories per day for your nutritional needs, you can't devour 4,000 calories every day- even if it's all salad!

So, yes, stop counting calories. But, no, don't eat unless you're actually hungry.

Fourth, treat carbs as potential toxins instead of quick energy

Finally, remember that carbs are not a source of quick energy (only). Rather, they're toxins. As such, your body will burn them using the WIFO (worst in = first out) rule of elimination. That will place you right back into sugar-burning mode where your body 1) eliminates sugar by converting the first batch to fast energy, then 2) converts what it can't immediately use to body fat.

You already know that, I know. So let me emphasize something else about your gut and the importance of the fuel you place inside of it.

Did you know that the gut is often referred to as your *second brain*? Your stomach and your gut have the same shape, they're comprised of the same tissue, and they each have their own nervous systems- each with millions of neurons.

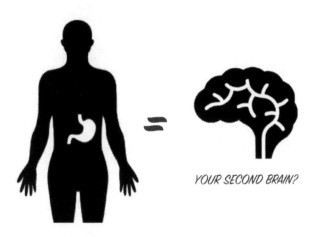

YOUR SECOND BRAIN?

Now, I realize you might not have known those few facts, but I guarantee that you've have insight- or intuition- and just *known* that something was *really* right or that something was a bit "off." How? Because *you knew it in your gut!*

Or, you stepped into the unknown. You were brave. You knew it was a stretch for you, some uncharted territory where you didn't know the outcome, and you had butterflies- read: doubts- in your stomach!

Here's what I'm driving at: your gut is important. In fact, gut health is one of the greatest factors determining your overhaul health and well-being. Here are a few of the important functions of your gut:

- Your immune system (80% of it!) is largely housed in the gut.

- Your cardiovascular health and many of your major organs are tied to the gut.

- Your gut's condition determines what your body can do with the nutrients you take in- including the nutrients you ingest from food and from supplements.

(By the way, I used to be the model of un-health, so I learned each of these the hard way. Take the short-cut and learn from my hard-earned experience.)

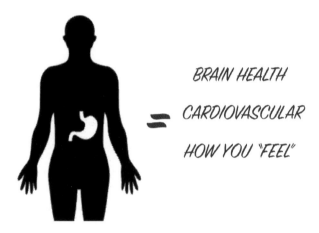

BRAIN HEALTH

= CARDIOVASCULAR

HOW YOU "FEEL"

Perhaps this helps you understand how people have been able to do things like:

- Treat cancer with dietary changes

- Lessen the effects of- or even heal- ADD & ADHD with dietary changes

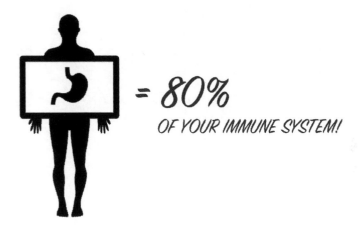

= *80%*
OF YOUR IMMUNE SYSTEM!

- Rebuild their immune systems with better nutrition[133]

The saying "You are what you eat" proves true.

(No wonder I was always cranky + tired + had joint pain + took a long time just to stand up out of the bed when I woke up in the morning + experienced MAJOR digestive issues every time I ate + ... *we don't even have time to go into all of it here.*)

I know. We eat on the go. We don't think much about what our stomachs need- other than "feed me" and move on...

I challenge you to go back the first two statements I made in the book. I've repeated them several times, so by now you may remember that 1) the causes of all dis-ease can be reduced to toxins and deficiencies, as well as 2) your body self-heals when you get those two factors in order.

I regularly teach health classes and receive the same question: "I'm way out of shape. How do I begin getting this in order?"

---

[133] "Eating or drinking too much sugar curbs immune system cells that attack bacteria. This effect lasts for at least a few hours after downing a couple of sugary drinks" (https://www.webmd.com/cold-and-flu/cold-guide/10-immune-system-busters-boosters#1, accessed 4-29-2018).

I always answer the same: "Start with your gut. Begin eating right. Before you ingest something, think about whether it's a toxin or a nutrient, whether it's harmful or helpful. If it's the first, don't eat it. If it's the second- and you're actually hungry- go for it."

And I remind them that 80% of your immune system is housed in your stomach. And 80% of how you look and feel depends on what goes into that stomach rather than the exercise you do.

During a supplements class I teach I also tell people to begin with the gut by taking a probiotic, even as they change their diet. I urge them not to begin by drinking protein shakes or ingesting loads of vitamins.[134] Here's why: if your body can't digest the nutrients, you'll just "poop out" what you're taking without receiving any nutritional benefit. In other words, you'll poop good money down the drain.

Though many of us have used our stomachs as dumping grounds for all kinds of garbage, the good news is that the body will regenerate. It will self-heal when you provide what it needs.

You can think + do different

I know. Some of this runs counter to what you've always known. I've just told you that-

- To eat for weight loss; exercise for strength & mobility

- To eat based on macros- not food "groups" or "pyramids"

- To stop counting calories, and just eat when you're hungry

---

134 See www.OverflowFaith.com/p/supplements (the domain is case-sensitive). Or, go to appendix C in this book.

- To treat carbs as potential toxins instead of quick energy

To get different results than you've gotten before, you'll need to adjust a few of the things you've historically done. That's right, *think + do different.*

In the following chapter we'll do a quick review. I'll remind you of what happens when you eat each of the macros we've studied. At this point we'll start putting all the pieces together.

In the chapter after that, I'll outline six benefits of Keto that go beyond weight loss. Then, finally, in the last chapter of the book I'll give you seven practical steps to getting started!

13. WHAT HAPPENS WHEN YOU EAT WHAT

MAIN IDEA: IT'S NOT JUST THE NUMBER OF CALORIES YOU CONSUME THAT'S IMPORTANT; THE KIND OF CALORIES YOU CONSUME MATTERS MORE.

This chapter contains a lot of review. If you begin reading a few pages into this one and think, "*Hmmm, I think I know this already*," great! That's intentional. I want to being putting all the pieces together, so that you're better equipped to reap the benefits of Keto.

A few chapters ago we compared your body to an engine- to a hybrid engine that can burn two types of fuel. You can burn carbs (i.e., glucose, sugar) or fats (including fat already stored by your body).

Let's take that a step farther...

Everyone agrees that the kind of fuel you put in your vehicle's engine matters. If the manufacture calls for diesel, that's what you "feed" the car. If you have a high performance hot rod, you opt for a higher octane fuel. In other words, all fuels are not created equal...

When I was in grad school I pulled into a gas station and, in haste, pumped my 1996 Pontiac Sunfire- an automobile I'd bought brand-spanking new just a few years earlier- with a *full tank* of diesel. Problem was... well... that little red sports car ran on unleaded fuel *only*. The diesel wasn't only unusable, if I'd cranked the car and pumped that fuel through the lines and into the carburetor, I'd have a massively expensive problem on my hands.

Thankfully, I realized what I'd done before turning the ignition. I pushed the car to the corner of the lot, let it sit there through the weekend, and then had it towed to a nearby garage as soon as it opened the following Monday morning.

It cost me $100 to have the tank emptied.

And I lost the entire tank of fuel I'd put in it.

And I still needed to buy gas.

Why?

Because all fuels aren't created equal.

The same thing is true of the fuel you put in your body. By now, you've seen that all foods aren't the same. In fact, I'd argue that some foods- the highly processed, lab-created versions- aren't actually foods at all. Your body responds to them the same way my beloved Pontiac would have responded to dumping a few liters of Mountain Dew into the tank.

How do you determine if it's good fuel?

Every time you eat (or drink) you consume calories. What those calories do- and how your body is able to use them- actually depends on the kind of calories they are. Your body converts all calories into *something* before it uses them.[135] When we evaluate what they do inside your body, that helps us determine whether or not it's good fuel source for us.

This is why it's a bad idea to just "count calories." A flawed nutrition strategy says, "I'll just eat less than I burn and I'll be fine. As long as I'm always spending more than I consume, I won't gain weight."

No worries if you've fallen prey to this line of thinking. It's exactly how most people have been conditioned to think about nutrition.

FLAWED NUTRITION / WEIGHT LOSS STRATEGY >>>

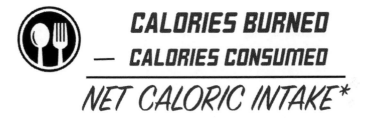

CALORIES BURNED
— CALORIES CONSUMED

NET CALORIC INTAKE*

*THE FLAW IS THAT WE ASSUME CONSUMING LESS THAN WE BURN AUTOMATICALLY CREATES WEIGHT LOSS!

At first glance, it sounds like this equation would work. And, in fact, it might have worked for you when you were younger- back when you weren't carb-sensitive and you weren't insulin-resistant.

If this equation was true, though… just think about it… that means you and I could go on an "Dr. Pepper and Baby Ruth" diet, right?

Let's work the math…

---

[135] *Bulletproof Diet*, p31.

A 20-ounce Dr. Pepper boasts 250 calories, and a full-size Baby Ruth contains 280 calories. If I have one of each for breakfast, lunch, and dinner, my caloric intake will be 530 calories per meal (250 + 280 = 530), or 1,590 calories per day (530 x 3 = 1,590). If I add another for a mid-afternoon snack- something I should easily be able to do for a 5'10" male that works out regularly and weighs around 170-175 pounds, I'll consume 2,120 calories that day. (Notice that this puts us right at the 2,000 calorie recommendation.)

Even though I burn far more calories than that, ironically, if I eat this meal plan for a week I'll likely *gain* weight!

Why? *Because all calories aren't created equal.*

Cattle farmers refer to "feed efficiency," a term used to denote how effective food is in putting weight on their animals. The goal, particularly when raising cattle and chicken, is to *plump them up even while feeding them less.* Thrifty farmers have learned that by giving estrogen to their cattle they can incite rapid weight gain with 30% *fewer* calories.[136]

That saves them money on the production-side. And, it creates a better bottom line.

(It's also another reason to eat grass-fed beef from a reputable source.)

Now, if adding a small amount of a single hormone to cattle feed can achieve this outcome, what might the multitude of factors affecting our foods do to our bodies? You see, **weight loss isn't just a matter of consuming less than you burn. On paper, the equation always makes sense, but your body is more complex than basic math, right?**

---

[136] *Bulletproof Diet*, p33.

So what do these fuels do?

So, by way of review, there are three possible fuels you can consume: carbs, protein, and fat. And, they each do three different things as they move through your body.

First, let's discuss carbs. All carbs (regardless of whether they come in the form of a carrot, a pizza, or a bowl of table sugar) do the following:

- **Glucose.** Carbs first convert to glucose and are used as "quick energy" by your body.

- **Glycogen.** You can only use a limited amount of quick energy, so the next approximate 1,600 calories of glucose are converted to glycogen and stored in your muscles. Note: if you already have some glycogen stored (most people do), you'll fill these reserves only.

- **Body fat.** Remaining glucose converts to body fat, where it is stored for "future use."

The exception to the above 3-step pathway for carbs is fructose (which is found in high concentration in fruits and is found in high fructose corn syrup). Fructose bypasses steps 1 & 2 and goes immediately to step 3!

By the way, a lot of people think the can't get through the day without "quick energy." But you don't nearly as much "quick energy" as you think. For instance a 30-minute run *might* burn 300 calories *if* you run with a steady pace. That's the equivalent of a candy bar. But the candy bar is junk fuel with a lot of fructose that doesn't convert to glucose- it bypasses this process entirely.

THE PATHWAY CARBS TAKE IN THE BODY >>>

1. CONVERTS TO GLUCOSE
A SMALL AMOUNT IS USED FOR THIS "QUICK ENERGY"

2. REPLENISHES GLYGOCEN
THE NEXT BATCH REPLENISHES GLYCOGEN STORES IN YOUR MUSCLES

3. STORED AS BODY FAT
MOST IS STORED AS "BODY FAT" FOR FUTURE USE!

Second, let's evaluate protein. The first thing to remember is that your body needs some protein- though probably not near as much as you'd think. In fact, it's super-easy to over-do it with protein.[137]

When you ingest protein, two things occur:

- **Biological needs.** Your body first captures what it needs to maintain bone density, muscle mass, etc. Because your body recycles protein, and because it conserves it, most people don't need as much protein as they think. In fact, most people overdue it!

- **Conversion.** Your body can't actually do anything with any extra protein you consume, so it gets rid of it through a process of *gluconeogenesis*.

There's that big word, again- the one I introduced in chapter 9. Let's review it. Remember, when we break apart the word *gluconeogenesis* we get an accurate mental picture of what the word means:

- *Gluco* = glucose

---

137 Remember, your body can recycle as much as 300 grams / day of protein.

- *Neo* = new

- *Genesis* = create

That is, your body creates new glucose from the protein overage. That means, in effect, that your body treats extra protein as if it is a carb, thereby sending it through the 1-2-3 step framework listed above.[138]

Third, let's consider fats. When you feed your body fats, your "shut off" the engine that burns carbs and you turn on the engine that burns fat for fuel. You body begins burning the fats you eat. Ketones are released as a byproduct and become the preferred source of fuel for your brain (which, remember, burns about 25% of your total daily calorie usage).

If your body needs additional fuel, it turns to the fat stored throughout your body, as it's in a "fat-adapted" mode. If you're not in a fat-adapted mode (read: you've been ingesting carbs), your body responds with hunger pains when there are no more carbs to consume. So, rather than burning your body's fat stores, you reach for something to eat and enter the carb cycle above of using quick energy and storing the remaining as body fat. **In general, if you eat fat you'll get thinner, if you don't eat fat you'll get thicker.**

In other words, here's the process for fats you consume:

- The body burns the food you consume, first (as long as carbs aren't present)

- After it's burned through the available food, your body begins using fat that's stored in your body for fuel (as long as you're in a fat-adapted mode)

---

[138] For a longer treatment of protein go to chapter 9.

What to expect as you make the transition to Keto

For most people, the transition from being a sugar-burner to burning fat is relatively easy. And, since your body only holds about 1,600 calories of glycogen in your muscles, many people make the transition in just a few days.

As I read websites and books and blog posts about Keto, many people warned of a 5-7 days of physical and mental frustration as your body made the switch from burning sugar to burning fat.

The repeated caution went something like this: "Beware of the first week or so. You'll likely feel an afternoon slump. You may feel a bit groggy and irritable. You might even get flu-like symptoms!"

Say, what? The flu!?

One author even referred to this feeling as "Keto flu."

I didn't experience that. For a day or so I felt a bit sluggish, but it wasn't overly dramatic. Plus, every time I felt a twinge of weirdness I simply realized that my body was feeling hungry, because it was craving more sugar. No, I wasn't always craving a Baby Ruth and a Dr. Pepper- I haven't had more than a handful of sodas in the past year, anyway. But, my body was craving the sugar found in french fries, cheese, yogurt, ice cream…

Since I expected this to occur, I wasn't surprised when it did. And, because of that, I knew exactly what I needed to do…

Like telling a toddler, "No, now is your bed time. You've got to be quiet and stop talking," I had to tell my body, "Whoa. Now it's time for this sugar-burning engine to shut down. Go to sleep, so the other engine can engage…"

Furthermore, I knew what you know now- that when that second engine engages, you'll *rarely if ever* feel hungry. The foods you eat will satisfy, plus your body will simply consume your body fat when you're *not* eating something.

Most people freak out at the first twitch of hunger. Just press on…

Rather than dealing with cravings and hunger pains, the biggest thing I noticed was this: *how many times I reach for carbs even when I'm not actually hungry at all!*

Before going Keto, I'd walk through our kitchen and grab a few crackers or handful of cashews- almost as if my body intuitively knew, "Hey, I'm going to need this in the next 30 minutes or so… might as well grab it while we're here."

Also, realizing how much I depend on food for nonsensical, emotional reasons was revelatory. Think about it: chocolate provides you with a quick dopamine hit- a legit sugar "high." *Feeling down or bored?* It gives you a boost… for just a few seconds.

These impulse grabs were, really, the only things I "missed" as I made the transition.

That said, here are two things you'll *physically* experience as you move to a Keto-based diet:

First, you'll begin burning body fat. In the first day or so, you'll burn through the glycogen that's stored in your muscles (your arms and legs will feel leaner, almost immediately). Around the second or third day, you'll feel the fat starting to go…

(By the way, generally, you'll see the belly fat starting to go first.)

Second, around the second or third day you'll also realize you have a *reduced* appetite. With your hunger hormones starting to balance, coupled with the fact that your body is receiving the nutrition it needs, you'll likely look at your watch one afternoon and think, "Hmmm... I haven't actually eaten yet. I really should grab something."

A few years ago people started proposing that we should eat 5 or 6 micro-meals throughout the day. The argument was that we weren't really created to eat "three squares a day," but that we were designed to munch throughout the day.

Turns out, *we weren't really designed to do either one.* Thousands of years ago it's unlikely everyone sat around the table at 7:00 am, 12 noon, and 6:00 pm. Nor did they grab something on-the-go by injecting two smaller meals at 9:30 am and 3 pm.

They probably ate once a day... *if they were lucky.*

Munching all day blasts your hunger hormones, keeps your blood sugar elevated, and insures you'll simply crave more food at shorter intervals. It creates a no-win situation in which you must *always* have food on hand.

Now, nutritionists have gone to the opposite extreme from the mirco-meal. They're writing about the benefits of intermittent fasting- of not eating after 8:00 pm in the evening and then allowing your digestive system to rest until late the following morning. (Some experts suggest you stop eating after 6:00 pm!)

I'm not advocating either one. On Keto, you eat if you're hungry. You don't eat if you're not. It's as simple as that.

How can I tell if I'm in ketosis?

That said, one way you can actually determine if your body is Keto-adapted (i.e., *fat-adapted*, burning fat instead of glucose) is if you can wake up and miss breakfast without feeling hungry until around 1:00 pm. If so, your body is sufficiently burning fat for fuel rather than depending on an influx of carbs and "quick energy."

(I know, I mentioned these earlier. It's great review, though.)

Another way to discern if you're burning fat for fuel is to evaluate how you feel after strenuous exercise. Were you able to complete the workout without having to eat beforehand? And were you able to continue for a few hours afterwards without feeling famished? If so, you're likely burning fat, as well, rather than depending on those "quick carbs."

At any rate, **within 4-5 days of "going Keto" you'll sufficiently have your hunger cravings under control and find yourself burning fat for fuel**. And, that's one of the primary goals of any weight loss strategy, correct?

People often ask me, *"How much will I lose?"*

Or, *"How fast will I lose it?"*

My disclaimer is *always*, "Well, that depends, every person is different, but…"

I continue, explaining that the average person has 4-5 pounds of extra water weight they're retaining in their muscles. Glycogen, that 1,600-plus calories of "stand by" energy that's comprised of the first reserved of unused glucose, holds a bunch of water. As a result, you can expect to urinate *a lot* during the first few days of Keto. If and when that happens, that's a good sign.

(Be sure to drink enough water- half your weight in ounces. For example, a 175-pound male should consume at least 87.5 ounces per day.)

After the initial dump of that 4-5 pounds of water weight during the first week, males will likely lose about 2 pounds per week and women will likely drop 1 pound per week. (I know, doesn't seem fair, does it?)

In addition, you'll begin to experience *the other benefits* of ketosis. Things like elevated energy levels and mental clarity. Things like improved memory and cognitive function.[139]

Why does this happen? Quite simply, your heart and your brain both "run at least 25% more efficiently on fat that blood sugar."[140]

And why does that happen? Well, it goes back to the concept we discussed at the beginning of this chapter: all fuels aren't created equal, and all calories aren't the same. When you provide you body with the good gas that it needs, well… things begin running far more efficiently and effectively.

And do you remember that bit we discussed about your body's ability to self-heal? Well, *this is that*, too. When you provide you body with the nutrients it actually needs, astounding things happen.

In the next chapter I'll outline seven benefits of going Keto (including weight loss), and you'll see just how good the fat fuel source is.

---

139 The book *Wheat Belly* discusses this in detail.

140 *Dr. Colbert's Keto Zone Diet*, p55.

14. SIX BENEFITS BEYOND WEIGHT LOSS

MAIN IDEA: YOU DON'T HAVE TO CHOOSE BETWEEN LOSING WEIGHT AND LIVING HEALTHY. WHEREAS SOME WEIGHT LOSS PROGRAMS CREATE HEALTH ISSUES, THE KETOGENIC PLAN OF NUTRITION BENEFITS YOUR BODY IN NUMEROUS WAYS IN ADDITION TO WEIGHT LOSS.

I used to cut *a lot* of weight. And I spent time with a bunch of other guys who did.

You see, when I was in high school I wrestled. An individual and team sport, wrestlers grapple with opponents based on weight classes. When I competed, teams consisted of 14 guys- one team member for each respective weight class. Our school wrestled against rival teams- each man going 1:1 with the foe of the same weight. Although the scoring scenario is a bit more complicated that I want to venture into here, the basic gist is that the team with the most individual wins is deemed the team winner.

As a wrestler, my goal was to compete in as light of a weight class as possible. I'd shed as much body fat as possible, dropping the pounds in order to challenge smaller opponents.

That's what we *all* did. Some of us cut a few pounds; some guys dropped 20 or more. Remember, too, we were *only* in high school, and we were *already* athletes who had been training most of the year. We didn't have a lot to lose, so much of what we lost was muscle and water weight.

We employed strange methods to lose the weight, too. Things like-

- Running 8-10 miles with trash bags under layers of sweat pants and thermal shirts- all in an effort to sweat more and lose water weight

- Starving- literally- for several days at a time

- Spitting to fill a 32-ounce cup, all in the hopes of "spitting out" weight (don't laugh, it works- and it goes even faster if you're chewing gum to make you salivate)

- Popping pills that make you poop or pee (again, short-cuts to chopping off pounds)

The result is that most of us looked gaunt. Our faces got hollow. We became tired, sluggish, and moody.

My kids' mother knew me in high school. We dated off and on. Even now, decades later, she'll tell you, "He was *nasty* during wrestling season. He turned into a completely different guy."

She's right. I did. I lost too much weight and I lost it in a way that mitigated *against* my health. It hurt me- it didn't help me.

Now, it's easy to look at the methods we used back then and label them as clearly *mad*. But, the truth is that many diet fats on the market today basically do the exact same thing:

- You over-exercise

- You starve

- You pop pills

- You eat nutritionally deficient foods

- You sacrifice vitality and life

In summary, you *exchange pounds for health!*

That's never a good trade. After all, **losing weight isn't just about looking good, nor is it only about feeling better. It's also about actually being physically healthy and whole.**

Over the next few pages, I'll show you six benefits of Keto *beyond weight loss*. You'll learn that the ketogenic diet is actively being used to treat, tend to, and manage *multiple* health concerns that have absolutely nothing to do with body weight at all. I'll demonstrate that **weight loss and health aren't at odds.**

(Plus, you might see a few ways to bless your friends and family by introducing them to Keto, too.)

WEIGHT LOSS SHOULDN'T REQUIRE UNHEALTHY CHOICES!

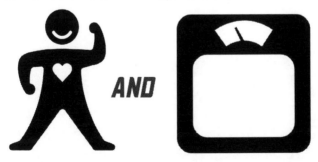

- YOU DON'T HAVE TO CHOOSE BETWEEN HEALTH & WEIGHT LOSS

Think about it like this: when you remove the toxins from your body (i.e., glucose) and replenish existing deficiencies by flooding your body with healthy nutrients (the fats your body needs), your body naturally gravitates to greater levels of health. To speak the language we used earlier in the book, **your body *self-heals* when provided with the nutrients it needs.** That self-healing includes better cognitive function, healthier emotions, increased energy, avoidance of a list of common health concerns, and- *yes!*- weight loss. **When healthy, your body moves towards its ideal weight *almost automatically.***

Here's where we're headed for the remainder of the chapter:

1. First, your brain prefers fat for fuel

2. Second, brighten your mood

3. Third, slow the aging process

4. Fourth, avoid issues caused by carbs

5. Fifth, feeling full > feeling hungry

6. Sixth, consistent flow of fuel = more energy

Of course, with Keto you'll also lose weight without going hungry, without growing tired, & without getting irritable- just like I promised in the subtitle of the book!

First, your brain prefers fat for fuel

The more I studied ketogenic nutrition, the more I was surprised to learn that **your brain works better on a high-fat diet than a high-carb diet.** One leading Keto authority writes,

> *"Ketones are actually the preferred fuel source for the muscles, heart, liver, and brain."*[141]

That is, these organs run *better* when fueled by fat rather than when fueled by sugar.

Now, I shouldn't have been surprised by this, because your body is going to run one of two fuel sources- fat or sugar. If your body is *not* burning fat, that means your body *is* fueling everything in your system with glucose (sugar), including your brain.

Look back at the quote: *your brain prefers ketones*. Ketones are the by-product of fat burning. So, when carbs are present and being burned, ketones are hardly used at all. On the other hand, although people worry about getting enough energy, when fat is being burned, carbs become irrelevant.

KETO BASICS

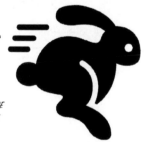

- YOUR BODY CAN RUN OFF GLUCOSE OR FAT.

- YOUR BODY WILL BURN GLUCOSE FIRST, BECAUSE OF YOUR BODY'S PROPENSITY TO ELIMINATE TOXINS FIRST.

- YOUR BODY WILL BURN FAT WHEN GLUCOSE IS NOT PRESENT, WHICH IS ITS PREFERRED FUEL SOURCE.

- YOUR BODY WILL STOP BURNING FAT AT ANY TIME GLUCOSE ENTERS THE BLOOD STREAM, THEREBY SHIFTING YOU BACK TO BEING A SUGAR-BURNER RATHER THAN A FAT-BURNER.

Remember the basics of Keto:

---

[141] *Keto Clarity*, p 35.

- Your body runs off either glucose or fat.

- Your body always burns glucose first, because of your body's propensity to eliminate toxins before anything else.

- Your body easily burns fat (it's preferred fuel source) when glucose is not present.

- Your body immediately ceases burning fat at any time glucose enters the blood stream, thereby shifting you back to being a sugar-burner rather than a fat-burner.

Your brain uses about 500 calories per day. When eating carbs, your brain "runs" on glucose, consuming about 120-125g every 24 hours (the equivalent of about 480 calories).[142] Ketosis transforms *your brain* into a fat-burning machine.

That sounds strange, I know. The reality, though, is that **your brain can't actually function on a low fat diet.** You see, your brain is 60% fat.[143] "Fat is also the basis for the lining of your nerves, called myelin, which allows electricity to flow efficiently. When you have more myelin, you literally think faster."[144]

Think back through the quick ketogenic history we reviewed earlier in the book. Keto was used over a century ago to treat epilepsy, a neurological disorder.[145]

---

[142] Carbs have 4 calories per gram.

[143] *Dr. Colbert's Keto Zone Diet*, p102.

[144] *Bulletproof Diet*, p43.

[145] See https://www.epilepsy.com/learn/about-epilepsy-basics/what-epilepsy for more about epilepsy. Accessed 4-28-2018.

Keto has also been used to treat ADD & ADHD. *That makes sense, doesn't it?* Fueling a kid's brain with sugar and processed foods simply throw gas on an already raging fire!

One of my sons is, let's just say... *impulsive.* He's busy.

Many of the issues he demonstrations related to attention-span and impulse control, I believe, can be tied directly to diet *and* activity. When we allow him to sit around and have lots of "screen time," his mind goes idle. Then, when we permit to ingest loads of sugar, we set him up for... let's just call them *neurological struggles.*

See what I'm saying?

This doesn't just effect kids, though. Let's face it. A lot of us adults fight to stay focused and keep engaged, don't we? How much of this is tied to sugar in our brains?

When I began Keto, my thinking *instantly* grew sharper and clearer. The mind fog lifted. The scattered feeling it's easy to get when you've got a lot going on... *gone.*

Now, I'm not against medication when it's needed. I am, however, against medication that's used to cover a symptom when we could address the body system itself and bring healing.

By the way, when you have time do a quick Google search on "Keto and Alzheimer's" and "Keto and Dementia." These are both cognitive issues that have some reversible conditions.

In addition, others have treated mental illnesses, including schizophrenia and bipolar disorder, with Keto. Still others have found relief from chronic migraines.

Why does this work? Because your body is *not* designed to run on sugar. When you opt to burn better fuel (fats) you reap better results.

Now, go back to the first two premises of the book:

- All dis-ease is caused by toxins and deficiencies, *and*

- Your body self-heals when it receives the nutrients it needs.

It puts some of these "brain" and "mind" issues in a different light, doesn't it?

Sure, your brain *still* needs *some* glucose (as do other parts of your body). When you're in ketosis, your brain will still "burn" glucose for about 25% of its needs. Turns out, though, your body can manufacture all the glucose it needs. And, when you're in ketosis, it will *only* manufacture what it needs and *nothing more.*[146]

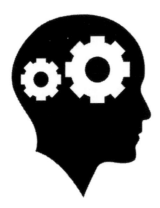

YOUR BRAIN

- *BURNS 500 CALORIES PER DAY*

- *IS 60% FAT*

- *PREFERS FAT / KETONES OVER SUGAR*

- *CAN'T FUNCTION ON A LOW FAT DIET*

- *CAN "REVERSE" CONDITIONS THAT ARE HARMFUL AND SELF HEAL WHEN TOXINS (I.E., SUGAR) ARE REMOVED AND NUTRIENTS ARE GIVEN*

---

146 We discussed gluconeogenesis in chapter 9 and chapter 13.

Second, brighten your mood

Depression is a mental health and wholeness issue, characterized by feelings of despair and hopelessness. Now, I'm definitely *not* suggesting a "sugar crash" is the cause of depression, nor am I equating the two. However, a sugar crash (experienced when your body is depleted of glucose and begins craving more) often elicits of sense of despair.

Think about it. A lot of mood swings are the result of feeling hungry and tired. If you can eliminate those two factors, you'll feel better- physically and emotionally. If you can keep your body from crashing, you can maintain your mood.

Turns out, there is no "crash" on Keto, as you have a constant supply of on-demand energy. That's great news.

Scientifically, the news gets even better, though. Ketones promote the production of Gamma Aminobutyric Acid (GABA), a brain chemical (neurotransmitter) associated with mood disorders.

- A lack of GABA is associated with depression and gloom
- GABA is an active ingredient added to anti-depressants

In other words, though I *am not* prescribing Keto as a cure for depression, I *am* implying that Keto is part of a holistic approach to health that includes both our *thoughts* (the first benefit of Keto mentioned in this chapter) and our *emotions* (the second benefit). Again, this depends on removing toxins and flooding your body with nutrients.

Also, let's be honest with each other…

A lot of our eating is strictly emotional, isn't it? We feel down, so we reach for the wine and chocolate. We have a long day full of hard conversations, so we grab the half gallon box of ice cream.

When you feel better, you can more readily cut that out. And that's a win on multiple fronts!

A BETTER MOOD = LESS EMOTIONAL EATING

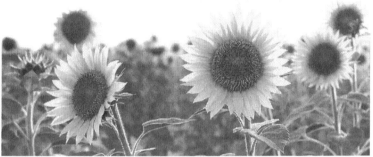

Third, slow the aging process

If you've ever exercised and then had sore muscles, you've experienced *oxidation*. That is, you've physically felt the process of your cells breaking down.

Here's the bad news. Oxidation happens every single day- just by living. Your cells require oxygen to function (notice the similarity between the words *oxygen* and *oxidation*), but that oxygen breaks your body apart:

> *"Oxygen in the body splits into single atoms with unpaired electrons. Electrons like to be in pairs, so these atoms, called free radicals, scavenge the body to seek out other electrons so*

they can become a pair. This causes damage to cells, proteins and DNA."[147]

Your cells are constantly strained, they consistently tear apart, and they regularly regenerate. And the free radicals which are released as a by-product of oxidation continue wreaking havoc.

The good news is that our cells rebuild themselves stronger than they were before. That's why you can lift weights for a few weeks in the gym, increasing your maximum lifts every few weeks.

But, *and this is a big deal...*

Over time, your cells don't rebuild as effectively- and those cells begin to look worn. In fact, some doctors suggest that aging is nothing more than the effects of oxidation multiplied over time.

AGING*

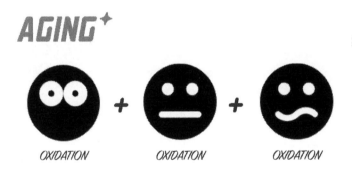

OXIDATION   OXIDATION   OXIDATION

* AGING = THE EFFECTS OF OXIDATION COMPOUNDED OVER TIME!

Let me provide you with a mental picture to help you understand what oxidation looks like in your body. Here you go: **oxidation is to your body what rust is to metal.**

---

[147] For more info, go to https://www.livescience.com/54901-free-radicals.html, accessed 4-28-2018.

Furthermore, in the same way that rusty pipes are full of corrosion and other issues that can be detrimental to the integrity of the pipe, the free radicals released in your body can cause a litany of issues:

> *"Free radicals are associated with human disease, including cancer, atherosclerosis, Alzheimer's disease, Parkinson's disease and many others..."*[148]

Got it? Yeah, I thought so...

Now, free radicals occur naturally: *"Free radicals are the natural byproducts of chemical processes, such as metabolism."*[149] Remember, your metabolism isn't just the rate of "how fast you burn calories," it includes all the processes your body requires to function. This means that the only way to *not* have free radicals is to *not* be alive. That's not really a good alternative, is it?

That said, there are two things you can do to help the situation.

First, you can stop adding extra free radicals to the mix. Turns out, two things increase the production of free radicals in your body more than anything else. And you have complete control over them. We've discussed them throughout this book:

- Sugar

- Processed foods

Which one of these will you not eat on Keto? Right, neither.

---

[148] For more info, go to https://www.livescience.com/54901-free-radicals.html, accessed 4-28-2018.

[149] For more info, go to https://www.livescience.com/54901-free-radicals.html, accessed 4-28-2018.

As a result, ketosis reduces the production of free radicals in your body. A side effect, then, is that you recover faster from exercise. And, of course, you slow the aging process.

Second, you can increase your intake of antioxidants. In the second part of the book I'll share with you my go-to for supplementation (appendix C).

Fourth, avoid issues caused by carbs

Glucose (sugar) doesn't just increase the release of free radicals into your body, it also causes several major health issues. When you "go Keto" you effectively avoid these other issues.

Earlier in the book we observed that our modern diet of sugar and refined carbs is responsible for "first world" health problems, including-

- Obesity

- Type 2 diabetes[150]

---

[150] Here's the difference between Type 1 and Type 2 diabetes:

Type 1 diabetes (often called "childhood diabetes," because that's when it's generally diagnosed) is marked by the body's inability to produce insulin. Recall, insulin is the key that allows the cells to open and receive glucose then distribute it throughout the body. Without an insulin shot, blood sugar can run high- even to lethal levels.

Type 2 diabetes (often called "adult diabetes") occurs when people become insulin resistant. The cause of this... is eating too much glucose, such that the body no longer responds to it. As a result, again, the blood sugar can run to abnormally high levels. Due to the dietary habits of the U.S., we are seeing a rise of Type 2 diabetes in children and young teens.

For more information go to https://www.webmd.com/diabetes/guide/types-of-diabetes-mellitus#2, accessed 4-28-2018.

- Heart disease, heart burn, and blood pressure

In the book *Dr. Colbert's Keto Zone Diet*, we find several other issues which many doctors connect to too much sugar in the diet.[151] Notably, Dr. Colbert reports (anecdotally) that people found healing for each of the following issues (this list is alphabetized):

- Aging slows down

- Arthritis

- Auto-immune improvement

- Chronic fatigue

- ED (Erectile Dysfunction)

- Fibromyalgia

- Hormone balance

- Irritable bowel syndrome

- Joints improve, aches eliminated

- Metabolic function restored

- Parkinson's

- Sleep disorders

- Type-2 diabetes- improved or healed

Now, it's interesting that most people actually agree, "Yes, eating less sugar helps all of those issues." However, most people don't make the correlation that your body treats carbs and sugar the exact same way

---

[151] *Dr. Colbert's Keto Zone Diet*, pp12-13.

once they hit your blood stream. Its like there's a mental "disconnect" here.

Jackie Eberstein, a noted ketogenic expert, says,

> *"Many chronic symptoms and health conditions such as fatigue, sleepiness, mood disorders, insomnia, gastroesophageal reflux disease, lipid disorders, high blood pressure, headaches (including migraines), gas, bloating, irritable bowel syndrome, joint inflammation, acne, and difficulty concentrating... will improve on a ketogenic diet.*
> ***Treating lifestyle conditions with lifestyle change such as this can make us a healthier and less drug-dependent country.***"[152]

In addition, others found healing from cancer. I know. It sounds strange that such a dreaded disease could be healed through diet. After all, we generally tackle this one with several rounds of chemotherapy- a method of treatment noted to be extremely harsh on the body.

Here's what the research shows, though:

> *"Cancers feed on sugars. Lowering or eliminating sugar intake [had] a direct effect on the cancer. The normal high carb, low fat diet of most people was simply feeding the cancers."*[153]

Again, **I want you to see these health benefits of Keto and uncover how others who don't even want to lose weight proactively use the diet to treat other conditions in the body.** As Dr. Fred Pescatore

---

152 Quoted in *Keto Clarity*, p63. Emphasis added.

153 *Dr. Colbert's Keto Zone Diet*, p6.

writes, "This isn't just some weight loss gimmick but rather a way to unlock your body's healing energy."[154]

Fifth, feeling full > feeling hungry

A few weeks into Keto I started reflecting on some of my eating habits. I remembered that I used to walk through our kitchen, grabbing a handful of trail mix or small stack of crackers with pimento cheese at specific intervals throughout the day.

I thought about it. *"Hmm... was this just habit?"* I asked myself.

Turns out, it wasn't. It was something different.

Now, I'm not discounting the fact that we can function *a lot* like Pavlov's dog. You know, we walk through the back door of the house after a long day and immediately pour ourselves something to drink- *automatically-* without thinking about it. Or we take a mid-afternoon break and *without even making a conscientious decision* meander to the snack machine, drop a few quarters in, and open a bag of *insta-carbs*.

That's *not* what was happening, though. Rather, I'd feel specific cravings for certain things.

- One day it was a banana.

- The next it might be a muffin, a bagel, or a piece of bread.

- The day after that it could be french fries, breakfast potatoes, or left-over tater tots.

---

154 *Quoted in Keto Clarity, p60.*

I discovered that my body craved "quick burn" energy, because was about to crash. As a result, it by default went into self-preservation mode before I even felt it. **Even when I didn't make a conscious decision as to what I wanted to eat, my body knew what it needed and instantly began reaching for it.**

Like I've mentioned a few times in the book, you're body doesn't have a dashboard with an "E" for empty and an "F" for full to gauge how much fuel remains in your tank. Hunger communicates that info to you.

But be clear: hunger is generally *not* telling you, "Hey, there's no fuel available."

Rather, hunger *most often* communicates, "I don't have any quick carbs. Fill me with something I can burn fast."

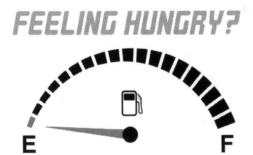

FEELING HUNGRY?

E   F

* *HUNGER IS GENERALLY NOT TELLING YOU, "HEY, THERE'S NO FUEL AVAILABLE. I'M STARVING!"*
* *RATHER, HUNGER MOST OFTEN COMMUNICATES, "I WANT QUICK CARBS. FILL ME WITH SUGAR!*
* *ON KETO YOUR BODY ADAPTS AND KNOWS YOU HAVE A CONSTANT FUEL SOURCE- YOUR BODY FAT.*

When you're eating Keto, though, your body adapts and knows you have a constant fuel source- *your body fat.* By paying attention to my body over the course of a few months on Keto, I've learned that the only times I actually feel hungry are when I've eaten a few carbs or sipped a sugary drink and- *as a result-* knocked my hunger hormones wonky (see chapter 8 for more).

Because "fat makes you feel full for longer periods of time more than anything else you could possibly consume," it's a natural appetite control. [155]

Sixth, consistent flow of fuel = more energy

So, yes, Keto "works in part by taking away your feeling of hunger."[156] When burning glucose (read: sugar), your body needs instant energy. *Consistently.* As a result, you constantly crave it. **Your body is smart and realizes that you're dependent on "just in time" fuel.**

As a result, you churn through quick energy all while continuing to store away the "slower" energy of fats. Yes, you read that right. You'll continue eating for fast energy even as your body stores away fat that could *readily* be used as "anytime" energy. It's the nutritional equivalent of begging for gas money to go to work every morning all while holding the keys to your own gas station.

To go Keto you must initially restrict your intake of carbs. However, it only takes a day or to to burn through the 1,600 calories of glycogen stored in your muscles. Once you use those reserves, your body will "flip" to the alternative fuel of fat.

Though you may experience a day-or-two long "crash," as long as you realize it's just a craving for sugar and nothing more (and that your body

---

[155] *Keto Clarity,* p86.

[156] *The Ketogenic Diet,* p240.

certainly won't starve because you have 100,000-plus calories of fat-fuel waiting to be used) you'll be fine. Within a few days you'll experience the benefits of on-demand, anytime energy.

While you make that shift, remember: **If glucose was a better source of fuel, you'd think that your body would convert unused glucose to "more glucose."** That is, it would just *keep* it. But it doesn't. It puts it in a form that your body can more readily use, a form that flows consistently as you need it.

If food you've recently eaten isn't available for energy, your body pulls from fat stores. Your "engine" is already "on" to burn fat (even if the fat has been stored for decades).

You'll experience natural appetite control, then, allowing you to go a long time between meals. Your body will constantly pull from the reserves it has. And, you won't get cranky when this happens. You'll feel better emotionally and have less mood swings- *not only* because of the presence of GABA in your system *but also* because you won't be hungry.

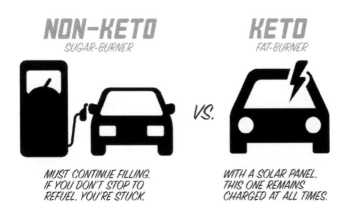

NON-KETO
SUGAR-BURNER

VS.

KETO
FAT-BURNER

*MUST CONTINUE FILLING.
IF YOU DON'T STOP TO
REFUEL. YOU'RE STUCK.*

*WITH A SOLAR PANEL.
THIS ONE REMAINS
CHARGED AT ALL TIMES.*

Since I began the Keto discussion by talking about engines, let's continue with that metaphor. Here's your comparison:

- **Non-keto, sugar-burner = gas**. If you're driving a gas guzzler, no matter how great your gas mileage is, if you don't refuel you'll find yourself stuck on the side of the road.

- **Keto, fat-burner = electric**. If you're driving an electric car with solar panels mounted to the roof, you have a constant supply of energy. You can go as long as you want to. You'll never run out.

Seventh, lose weight without going hungry, without growing tired, & without getting irritable

Finally, let's state the obvious. **You can- *and will-* lose weight on the Keto diet.** That's probably why you've read this book this far, right? You want to drop some unwanted baggage.

As you consistently eat Keto...

- Your thinking will be sharper + clearer

- Your mood will go up (which means you'll do far less emotional eating)

- You'll slow- and perhaps even reverse- the aging process

- You'll automatically avoid the long list of issues caused by carbs (while likely experiencing some degree of healing)

- You'll feel pleasantly full and won't go hungry (because your body will consistently use stored body fat as fuel)

- You'll always have energy

That said, the entire point of the chapter is this: **You don't have to sacrifice your health in order to lose weight.** It's not an either-or proposition whereas you choose weight loss at the expense of doing damage to some other area in your body.

Ready to get started?

Great. In the next chapter I'll tell you how...

15. GETTING STARTED

MAIN IDEA: YOUR NEXT STEP IS TO ACTUALLY BEGIN KETO. IN THIS CHAPTER WE'LL OUTLINE SEVEN SIMPLE STEPS TO HELP YOU START- AND CONTINUE- THE JOURNEY.

So you've hung with me for 200-plus pages. **At this point it's obvious that you either really, really love to read or you're ready to take the leap and "go Keto."**

By now, you know… plans that aren't implemented simply remain ideas. Even if they're good ones. **To get results you've got to take action. Over the next few pages we'll outline seven steps you can take now in order to begin.** Some of these will be things *you can do right now before you even finish the book.*

1. First, decide what you what to achieve

2. Second, pick a start date- *now*- even before you have all the info

3. Third, make a list of foods you will eat & foods you won't eat

4. Fourth, make predetermined decisions now for success later

5. Fifth, learn to read food labels

6. Sixth, prepare for mental road blocks and mindsets

7. Seventh, continue gathering resources

After reading these steps you'll be in a position to begin Keto *immediately*.

First, decide what you what to achieve

Before starting Keto you need to decide what you're trying to achieve. Most people go Keto in order to lose weight, then find themselves pleasantly surprised by the other benefits (see chapter 14). If weight loss is your goal, go ahead and decide how much you'd like to drop!

But go one step farther. **Your commitment should include *both* what you want to see happen *and* how long you're committed to this specific plan of eating**.

Here's why it's important to commit to a time period: *you will plateau at some point*. Don't be surprised when it occurs. Just realize that it's a temporary pause in your progress, and that your body will self-heal towards your ideal weight as you continue eliminating toxins and replenishing it with nutrients.

I remember "getting stuck" a few times during my own weight loss journey. Seems like it happened every 5-6 weeks, in fact. Part of my routine was that I weighed myself every morning- *at the same time-* which is something I emphatically suggest you do. Doing so helps you see your progress and teaches you how to make connections between your daily actions and the results you see.

I remember jumping on the scale one Tuesday and seeing the exact same number as the day before. It was frustrating. But, I stayed on my plan...

Then I weighed almost half a pound *more* on Wednesday. I wanted to quit.

(Now, mind you, I had already lost 25 pounds in just a few months. Despite that, one minor setback and I was ready toss in the towel!)

I maintained my composure, kept the routine, and weighed in the following morning. I weighed the exact same thing as the previous day!

Then something strange happened. On the following day I weighed *almost three pounds less.*

I *still* have no explanation for this. My best guess is that I had retained water-weight- or something odd like that. Then, a few days later, my body just "dumped it." I really don't know what happened.

I do know, though, that I didn't actually "lose that three pounds" overnight. Rather, it was the result of *consistent* actions that were taking me in the *right direction.*

Face it. Every day isn't going to be a great day. No worries. Stick with your plan. Trust the process, and everything will work out in the end. I guarantee it.

That said, you need to know the following:

- How much weight do you want to lose?

- How long are you committing to this plan, even if you don't see the weight fall off as quickly as you'd like to see?

(By the way, people ask all the time how much weight they can expect to lose on Keto. My default answer- *again*- is that you'll likely lose 4-5 pounds during the first week, particularly as your body dumps the glycogen stores and water weight they hold. After that, men generally lose about 2 pounds per week; women most often lose 1.)

Second, pick a start date- *now*- even before you have all the info

After deciding what you want to achieve (and how long you'll stick with it), your next step is to select a "go date." **Ideally, choose a day that's within 3 days from now. Don't put it off.** There will always be a birthday, holiday, wedding, or some other event that will potentially interfere with Keto. Plus, once you see what foods are friends vs. foes you can pretty much navigate any food situation (especially when you're not hungry all the time!).

Don't rationalize with something like, "I'll start after I finish the chips, cookies, or the bowl of ice cream."

And don't do the "I'll wait until New Year's" thing- *unless New Year's is next week.*

When I began my weight loss journey, it was the beginning of March. My New Year's resolution failed miserably, so I just began on a random Sunday (it was a Friday evening when I made the decision to start).

How do you begin Keto?

Great question. I've heard of two ways to begin. Let me tell you what they are, then explain them, then give you my recommendation.

- **Option 1: Taper down the carbs and "work your way into Keto."** Some proponents of the low-carb diet suggest you begin by cutting out *some* carbs. They suggest removing breads and other grains from your diet for a week. Then removing fruit. Then removing all sugars. Over the course of a few weeks, with a systematic plan, you'll find yourself at the "net 20 grams" Keto threshold.

- **Option 2: Cold turkey start.** Others suggest you go "all in" from the beginning, that you pick a go date and cut all the carbs.

WHICH WAY IS THE BETTER WAY TO START KETO?

OPTION 1 >
GRADUALLY CUT CARBS

OPTION 2 >
"COLD TURKEY"

- IT DEPENDS ON HOW FAST YOU WANT TO START BURNING FAT

Here's my suggestion: go "cold turkey."

Now let me tell you why. Carbs hijack your hunger hormones, right? And carbs in your system keep your body from burning fat. So why wait to go all in? Why endure the wonky hunger pains that carbs *will* produce? Why keep the extra glucose in your system- all the while knowing that you want to go Keto and shift your body to being a fat-burner instead of a sugar-burner?

In my opinion, **it's not worth the delay. If you're going to do the diet, go ahead and commit. You postpone your results by merely tapering down the carbs**. Go ahead and cut them out and reap the rewards.

Third, make a list of foods you will eat & foods you won't eat

I thought Keto would severely cramp my eating style. I thought, *Gee, once I go Keto I'll be stuck eating eggs, beef, and guacamole.* Throughout my research an interesting fact presenting itself: *the average person eats the same 30 foods over and over.* In other words, most of us already have a cramped eating style. If anything, Keto expands your horizons!

I've got two suggestions for you.

First, make a list of 40 foods that you can eat on Keto. Don't know where to start? Go to section A in the appendix. I've actually listed some "friends" and "foes" for you in section B.

Second, make a list of quick "go to" items that can grab at each meal. In the next step I'm going to encourage you to make some more predetermined decisions about foods in general. For now, let's just do that with the three main meals. It's great to have a few things in your mind already so that you don't ever feel "stuck" without any options. If you feel trapped, you're more likely to fail. Set yourself up for success.

For instance, though I'm not usually hungry at breakfast time, I know I can grab bulletproof coffee, an omelet, or leftovers from dinner the night before. (And I know I won't eat cereal, oatmeal, or a bagel.)

For lunch, I generally opt for a large salad with some sort of protein on it (i.e., grilled chicken, deli meat). This is an important point to note. On Keto you *won't* eat stack of bacon or long links of sausage. Rather, you'll eat 2-6 cups of salad each day and 1-2 cups of veggies (more than a lot of vegetarians). Fats are more dense nutritionally, so you won't need as much "fat" food.

For supper, I eat whatever the family eats. Sometimes I set bread to the side or eliminate the croutons from a salad, but since a few carbs are permitted on Keto, I don't sweat it. We all eat fairly healthy anyway.

One quick tip: **Keto becomes easier if you prep some of your food before hand.** For example, it takes no more effort to hard boil a full dozen eggs than it does to boil one, so go ahead and prep the entire tray. That way you have them for the week.

Or purchase a veggie tray whenever you make a grocery store run. We grab about two of these each week, set them on the kitchen counter, and let the kids graze whenever they're hungry. I grab my fill, as well. Since we have nutritious food on hand, we don't easily swerve towards unhealthy options. A little planning sets you up for long-term success.

Fourth, make predetermined decisions now for success later

A few years ago, when I first decided to drop the extra weight during the mirror-incident in Hawaii, I made some predetermined decisions as to what I *would* do and *wouldn't* do going forward. For instance...

- I decided my Starbucks froo-froo drink had to go. Since I self-righteously blamed a ton of my heft on it, I kicked it to the curb.

- I decided I wouldn't eat any sandwiches for lunch- because of the bread. Instead, for every lunch I would order a salad as my main dish, and add a meat of some sort to it.

- I decided I would say "no" to any and all desserts that were offered to me, including birthday cake at parties.

- I decided I would stop drinking sodas and sweet tea, that I would drink water with every meal.

- I decided I wouldn't eat chips, candy bars, or anything you could buy in a snack machine. In fact, I decided I wouldn't snack at all.

There were a few more decisions, but you get the idea. **Though this list may look confining to you, it was *freeing* to me.** You see, I knew I would face all of these situations every single day almost by default. **By making the decision *now*- and by making it *once*- it freed me to enjoy the day without wondering, "What will I do when _____ is offered to me?"**

In my previous *failed* weight loss attempts, I learned that walking into a meal without a plan always proves more difficult. Or facing a birthday cake without an answer can get awkward. It's easy to rationalize, and it's easy to negotiate with yourself. Especially when it's all in your head and no one else knows.

Plus, I discovered that "will power" is an exhaustible resource. If I'd endured a particularly long day at work (or even at home with the kids), I found myself battling *decision-fatigue*. I definitely knew when I'd gotten

to the end of my capacity to make a good choice. Or to make any
choice at all. And that's when my will power usually caved.

You've likely been there, too. In fact, it's documented that when we're
tired and temptation presents itself, we're less likely to make good
decisions. Think about it-

- *Decision-fatigue* is why you can do great *all day* on a diet,
  only to "lose it" at 9:00pm.

- *Decision-fatigue* is why you can go out to lunch with a
  friend on Friday- after an entire *week* of successful dieting-
  and then crater when the waiter brings the dessert tray.

**The best time to make a decision about what you'll eat or not eat is
now- when you're not hungry and when there's no food on the
table.** Furthermore, coupling predetermined decisions with healthy
hormones (no carbs hijacking them, like we discussed in chapter 8) and
satiety (full on fats) sets you up for success. Of course, reminding
yourself of your results- the progress you continue to see- helps, too.

*What are some more examples of decisions you might make now for
success on Keto?* Here are a few more of my own- particularly as to
what I do when I'm eating out. Eating at home is easy- you have
complete control over the menu. Going out, though requires some
forethought. This one's important to grapple with- 1/3 of calories come
from restaurants, according to FDA.[157]

Here's what I do- and what I suggest you try:

- Skip the appetizers, including the bread or chips you're
  offered.

---

[157] Source: FDA.gov/food/ingredientspacking/labeling/labelingnutrition/ucm248732.htm

- Steer clear of sugary drinks at coffee shops- and opt for heavy cream rather than half-and-half (no soy, either).

- Order the fajitas at the Mexican restaurant- give the rice, beans, and tortillas to one of your kids and skip the chips. Load up with as much sour cream and guacamole as you want.

- Drink water instead of tea, sodas, and sugary juices. In fact, commit now to *not* drinking your calories unless it's a special occasion (i.e., a glass of red wine).

- Trade the pile of rice at the Indian restaurant (my wife's favorite food!) for steamed vegetables. It's not an option on the menu, but I've never been to a restaurant that doesn't gladly make the swap.

- Forced to eat fast food? Grab a salad. Put grilled chicken or fajita beef on it. (You can do the same thing when everyone goes out for pizza.)

- If they don't have salad but serve hamburgers (i.e., Five Guys), opt for a lettuce wrapped cheeseburger. Feel free to add bacon and mushrooms, but skip the fries.

- Trade potatoes, corn, carrots or other carb-mongers for asparagus, spinach, or something else that's green when presented with those options as side dishes. I do this when I'm with my girls at the Cheesecake Factory on our monthly date night.

- Decide now about dessert. In general, the answer should be "no." I, however, I have one exception…

STAYING ON KETO

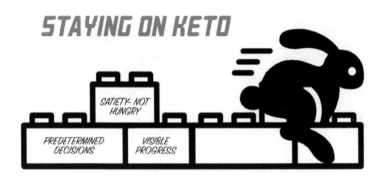

My favorite dessert *in the entire world* is white chocolate bread pudding. Especially when it's paired with ice cream. I could literally eat it by the platter.

But... you know where this goes... it's definitely *not* Keto-friendly. Nothing about it is. The bread is one big carb. The ice cream is nothing but sugar. And the entire dish is basked and then baked with more sugar.

But I still really, really like it.

So here's what I do. I've made a decision that whenever I visit a new restaurant that has bread pudding of any kind, it's fair game for me. I've already decided that I will order it and then relish *two* exquisite bites. That's it. That's my limit. *Two bites.* Then, I send the dish around the table for everyone else to enjoy.

I've discovered that plowing through the entire dessert delivers me no more satisfaction than two slow, savored bites. Those two bites provide me with the taste that I crave, they allow me to evaluate whether or not this restaurant's bread pudding is on par with the others I love, and I don't feel guilty (or bloated) after pounding away 700-plus calories of sugar.

Plus- and this one is huge, too- it always creates a fun moment for the entire table. We all share the food, we all laugh about the two bite max (of course, there are always a few people who break it!), and we're all a little better for the entire experience.

If you've got a sweet tooth, don't declare cheat *day*. Don't even declare a cheat *meal*. You'll lose valuable progress. Rather, make a cheat bite. Or two. It works great for me.

Fifth, learn to read food labels

We discussed these in chapter 6. **It's super-important that you learn to the food labels, since the entire premise of Keto is based around the 80-15-5 ratios of fats-protein-carbs.**

In order to get the ratios right in your diet, you'll need to recognize them on the foods you eat. No worries, though. The information isn't hard to find as *all prepackaged foods are required to have them*. And, since the government standardizes them, *they all look the same*. Once you know what you're looking for, deciphering the info becomes extremely easy.

In addition, even though restaurants *are not* required to publish the information, in our day of savvy consumers who hyper-share everything on the Internet, most establishments make it extremely easy to find their nutritional info both online and in the establishments.

Here's what you have to watch for, though: **most restaurants are still more concerned about the calorie count than the macro-makeup of the food** (because that's what most people are concerned with). Many of them post the info directly on their menus or in the advertisements for the food.

If they share more "surface level" information like the calorie count, they generally tell you whether something is "low fat" or not. By now you're super-smart about that and know the truth- if the fat has been removed from something sugar has been injected into it in order to make it taste right. Do a little digging on the website of the restaurant you're looking for and they'll generally provide you *all* of the information that's on the FDA food labels.

TARGET RATIOS, ASSUMING 2,000 CALORIES/DAY

	% OF DIET	CALORIES	GRAMS
FATS	80%	1,600	178
PROTEIN	15%	300	75
CARBS	5%	100	25

Let me give you a great activity you can do right now that will help you learn to read the labels while taking a step forward on your Keto journey. **Go rummage through your pantry and clean it out.**

First, place the following items on your kitchen table:

- Alcohol (except red wine)

- Anything you bought that came in a box (chips, snacks, cereal) unless it was specifically purchased as Keto-friendly

- Artificial-everything (including, but not limited to sweeteners)

- Candy

- Dried fruit, including raisins, "craisins," and shriveled peaches

- Fruit juices, including apple and orange juice

- Honey

- Jelly & jam

- Low fat *anything & everything*

- *Obvious carbs (i.e., potatoes, bread, bagels, muffins)*

- Sodas

- Sports drinks (like Gatorade, Powerade, etc.)

- Sugar and artificial sweeteners

- Syrups

- Sauces & condiments

- Some veggies (carrots, yams)

- Unhealthy oils (margarine, soy, soy bean oil)

- Wheat, grains, beans

Second, review the food labels on each of these items, noting only the number of carbs, grams of protein, and total fats. Doing this will help you see patterns and start categorizing food based on macros.

(Remember, the actual carb count is the total carbs *minus* the fiber.)

Third, toss it all in the trash. Or, if you feel bad about tossing it in the trash, give it away.

Sixth, prepare for mental road blocks and mindsets

I've fasted for extended periods a few times. About the second or third time I did, I noticed something strange about my mindset: *there was a huge mental block that occurred the first few days.* Since I knew I was going without food for a week or so, and since I believed I *should* feel hungry and weak, I actually did... *even though I wasn't.*

Let me explain.

My morning exercise routine consists of something like this:

- Wake up

- Walk to our bathroom, where I use the restroom, change into my workout clothes, and brush my teeth

- Go downstairs, drink a few ounces of water

- Head out the back door to the gym or simply begin running as soon as I get to the street

That's it. I'm literally in motion *within 15 minutes or less of waking up*. There's no breakfast, there's no hydrating myself, there's no mental prep or stretch... I just move right into it. And I feel really good stepping right into that routine.

When I choose to run, I generally take the first mile pretty slow. I shift my weight around, swing and stretch my arms, and get my blood flowing. Once I'm warm, I significantly speed up.

Three years ago I got to the "speed up" part of the run and thought, "Oh, I don't feel strong today. I feel weak." Then- "It must be because I'm fasting."

Here's the issue with that line of reasoning, though: it was *the first day* of my fast. I ate the night before, and it's my normal routine- even when I'm not fasting- to simply head out the back door without eating. In other words, to that point my routine wasn't any different than on a normal day. It was all in my head, in other words.

The same thing happened the first time I tried Keto. I went to the gym for an interval work out. High intensity. In the back of my mind I thought, "Well, I probably won't have much quick energy today... because I'm not eating carbs."

What?!

I never carb load anyway on any day before I go to the gym. *Ever*. I just go and do my thing.

I'm communicating this to you so you know to expect some mental pushback:

- Expect to feel weak the first day

- Expect to feel some sort of sugar-detox that feels like the "Keto flu"

- Expect a few hunger pains

- Expect to feel a little big sluggish

- Expect some of it to be real and expect some of it to just be in your head

And then flood your mind with the positive side of things, "Oh, yeah, I'm doing a great work right now. I'm transitioning my body from burning sugar to burning fat. This feels awkward for the moment, but it's going to feel really great in just a few days. **I knew this mental hurdle would come. No surprises here. So, I'm going to push right through it.**"

By the way, for some early motivation jump on the scales the night *before* you start Keto. Then go a few days on the diet. On the fourth or fifth morning, weigh yourself. Note the progress you've made.

What will you see? Again, you'll likely drop 4-5 pounds during that first few days, particularly as your body dumps the extra water weight that hold the glycogen stores in your muscles. Your clothes will already feel looser, you'll have more energy, and you'll have sufficient motivation to continue.

Seventh, continue gathering resources

Finally, as you move through the first week, continue gathering resources to assist you on your Keto journey. Here's what I've done.

First, get an app on your phone that does the mental work for you. I downloaded a non-ketogenic-specific app on the iTunes Store called *Lose It!*, which allows me to track macros and enter my body weight every few days. I don't have to count the carbs, protein, and fat grams myself- *the app does it all*. Nor do I even have to know how many grams *of anything* are in the foods I regularly eat. Again, that app already has them entered.

(This allows me to check a food before I decide to eat it or not, also.)

Second, download a few podcasts. And shake it up. Don't just download Keto-only podcasts, look for some alternatives that promote the low-carb lifestyle. In this book I've provided you with a 30,000 feet high overview of Keto. On the podcast feed you'll find niche discussions about each of the macros, dealing with specific health issues, using Keto for your kids or aging parents, and dozens upon dozens of other specific questions you may have. Expanding your horizon will help you determine how to best make Keto work for you.

Third, read a few more books. Sure, the basics of Keto are the same regardless of who you read. But, in my research I discovered that some authors major on some issues and minor on others, whereas other writers do the exact opposite. A variety of perspectives helps- as everyone speaks the same truth in a unique voice that helps us clarify the message even more. I've listed a few of my favorite books and websites in appendix D.

Fourth, supplement your nutrition. The first reason is this: you and I can never, ever eat enough to provide our body with all the nutrients it needs. In appendix C I outline the specific products I use every single day. They're the absolute best place to begin.

(You can also view the supplements class at www.overflow.org/p/supplements. Note: the webpage is case-sensitive; go *all lower-case* when you type it into your web browser.)

Fifth, finally, go to the resource page for this book. You'll find it at FindingKeto.online. On that page you'll find:

- The audiobook of this book
- Videos explaining Keto in simple, everyday language

- Links to articles and other helpful resources to empower you to continue this journey

---

Back full circle

This leads us back to where we began, to one of my core convictions: **your body is self-healing. That is, your body's natural state is actually health. When you offer your body the nutrients it needs- and remove the toxins it doesn't need, your body does an incredible job, almost effortlessly, of moving you towards greater wholeness.**

I guarantee...

- Your thinking will become sharper, your mood will elevate.

- Your youth + vigor will renew, as the aging process slows or even reverses.

- You'll overcome health issues with which you've struggled for years.

- You'll stop feeling hungry, all while feeling more energetic.

And, *yes*, you'll lose weight fast without going hungry, without growing tired, and without getting irritable.

PART 2 | YOUR PLAN & PRACTICAL TIPS

A. KETO-FRIENDLY VS. KETO-FOE FOODS

MAIN IDEA: MOST PEOPLE EAT THE SAME 30 FOODS OVER AND OVER. IF YOU CAN IDENTIFY 40 "GO TO" FOODS FOR KETO, YOU'LL NEVER BE STUCK WONDERING WHAT YOU CAN EAT, THEREBY SETTING YOURSELF IN A BETTER POSITION FOR SUCCESS.

When I began the Keto diet, I thought my food intake would become radically restricted. Turns out, the opposite happened. Throughout my studies I learned that-

> *"Data on food consumption show that people eat about thirty different foods on a regular basis, cycling through them all in about four days."*[158]

In other words, although we think that a diet or eating plan might constrain us, the reality is that we already live that way anyway. If anything, a new eating plan will expand your horizons.

---

[158] *The Ketogenic Diet*, p7.

In this chapter we'll identify several foods that are great "go to" options for Keto, as well as make a short list of things you'll likely bump into every day that you should simply push to the side.

Keto-friendly

Avocado (or guacamole)

Bacon

Beans

Butter

Cream

Cheese

Condiments like sour cream, salsa, and hot sauce

Eggs

Fish & other seafood

Green vegetables (like broccoli, kale, spinach, and other leafy greens, as well as celery and asparagus)

Heavy cream

Hot drinks like coffee and tea- don't add sweeteners

Meats, including sliced meats and deli meats

Milk substitutes- like almond milk or coconut milk

Mushrooms

Nuts

Oils

Peanut butter (or alternatives like almond butter, just read the label first)

Poultry (not fried)

Protein shakes (verify the carb count first)

Raw vegetables

Salad

Tofu

Keto-foes

Bread

Candy

Chips (unless specified as Keto-friendly)

Crackers (unless specified as Keto-friendly)

Corn

Dried and dehydrated fruits

Flour

Freeze-dried fruits (like bags of strawberries or blueberries which are often used to make smoothies- they had the water removed, leaving a high concentration of sugar)

Fruits which are high in sugar (i.e., bananas, grapes)

Grains (rice, oats, etc.)

Honey

Jellies & jams

Juices

Milk (skip the 2%, 1%, skim, soy, and half-and-half versions- opt for heavy cream)

Pasta- of all varieties, shapes, and sizes

Potatoes (i.e., baked potatoes, sweet potatoes, French fries, hash browns, etc.- these are all starches)

Sodas

Soy

Sports drinks

Sugar (including sugar using other names like "cane" or "syrup")

Sugar substitutes

Syrup(s)

Trail mixes (and even nut mixes- because they generally have a high percentage of hidden carbs in the form of candy and dried fruit)

Words you can't pronounce (generally ingredients ending in "ose," such as dextrose, sucrose, etc.)

B. SURPRISES

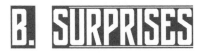

MAIN IDEA: YOU'LL BE PLEASANTLY SURPRISED BE SOME OF THE FOODS YOU CAN EAT ON KETO, AND YOU'LL BE SHOCKED BY SOME OF THE ONES YOU CAN'T.

I was shocked by a few of the things I learned were Keto-friendly as opposed to things that were Keto-foes. In this brief chapter, I'll highlight a few of the surprises.

- Breakfast foods like oatmeal, pancakes, waffles, and pastries contain a super-abundance of carbs

- Carrots, corn, potatoes, sweet potatoes = high carbs (they're all starches, so they'll sabotage your progress)

- Eggs are a great option for any meal (scrambled, hard-boiled, as an omelet, any way you choose)

- Fruits are generally high in sugar- vegetables are a better snack option or side dish (dried fruits are even worse!)

- Grains are all generally extremely high in carbs

- Heavy cream is the best "go to" for your coffee. Milk and half-and-half both contain added sugar

- Most things that are "breaded" - fried, floured, "cakes," "nuggets," and "sticks" = loaded with carbs

- Red wine = 5g carbs per class only (well within the daily carb limit), and is a great alternative to beer and other forms of drinking

- Yogurt generally has a high carb count- so read the label

C. THE BEST VITAMINS & SUPPLEMENTS FOR KETO

MAIN IDEA: A FEW KEY SUPPLEMENTS CAN GUARANTEE YOUR BODY RECEIVES THE NUTRIENTS IN NEEDS, HELPING YOU REACH A PLACE OF OPTIMAL HEALTH.

I spent six months reading several books, scouring numerous websites, and listening to countless podcasts about the ketogenic diet as I began eating Keto. Over and over, leading authorities continued recommending similar kinds of supplements:

- A multi-vitamin or green supplement

- Fish oil (to supply omega-3 fatty acids)

- Probiotics (for gut health)

- Potassium

Over the next few pages I'll introduce you to these "Core 4," as I call them- plus a few more. I recommend that everyone take advantage of the four I discuss in detail. Then, if there are others your feel your body needs, add them to your regimen.

(Note, too, that over the next few pages I'll repeat some of the info we've covered in the book. It's intentional, as it helps you review the facts while seeing how they fit into the bigger picture of supplementation.)

Food is important, but even good food isn't enough

I learned that eating was the biggest factor in my weight loss- *not exercise*. And it's been the biggest factor in maintaining my health and fitness even post-weight loss. Right now, I'm at my ideal weight. Even at this point, though, **eating right has more to do with how I look and feel than exercise does.**

That may fly against everything you've been taught. But, think about it like this: even though my 7-mile run *may* burn 700 calories...

- If I drink Venti white chocolate mocha from Starbucks on the way to work in the morning, and I've replenished all of those calories with junk fuel that adds weight to my body even though it's unusable for nutrition.

- If I eat a slice of cheesecake from the Cheesecake Factory one evening while out with my girls (that's their favorite restaurant), my run is *done* plus I've consumed 300 *additional* calories.

- If I drink the large lemonade from Chik-fil-A (plus the obligatory refill), I tally the same number of calories and sugar load as that Starbucks drink.

The biggest factor for me is what I eat, not what I do. The same is true for you.

In other words, both diet and exercise are important. But, it seems that diet is the most important.

All that said, here's another lesson I learned. And it's the subject that we're diving into now: **even eating right isn't enough to fuel your body's nutritional needs. Good food is not enough.**

Over the next few pages I'll outline a few of the "must have" products you need to fuel your body- *particularly if your "fed up" with the status quo and want to move to greater levels of health.*

MultiGreens

MultiGreens is a green, plant-based supplement- packed with nutritional foods like kale. One of the main reasons you need a "green," food-based supplement is because... well... *who really eats enough greens?*

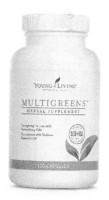

There are other reasons, too. Even if you do eat a lot of vegetables, other factors come into play...

- The dirt your food grows in isn't pure.

- Farmers often pick the food too early- before it's really ripe and ready to eat.

- Your food travels from where it's harvested to where you eat it. Most food loses a large percentage of its nutritional value within 8-16 hours of being picked. Since most of us don't eat "farm to table," our food takes weeks to travel from the farm to the warehouse to the larger warehouse to the truck to the grocery store and into our home.

- Your food is then stored, losing its "life" while in hibernation.

- Your food is cooked (it's entirely possible to "cook off" the remaining nutrients).

FARM TO TABLE?

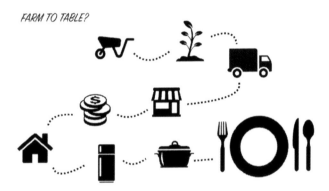

Core idea 1: The basic causes of dis-ease

The process above leads us directly into one of the core concepts of health. Basically, **all dis-ease in the body can be traced to two main causes:** *toxins and deficiencies.*

A toxin is something that should *not* be present in your body. Or, it's something that should be present, but it gets dangerous when it's present in too high of a quantity. Toxins include things like sugar, synthetics, and even stress. Our body can handle any of these in small quantities, but too much can literally be lethal.[159]

A deficiency, on the other hand, is when your body lacks something that *should* be present- when something that you need to support your body's systems isn't present in great enough quantity. For example, we need a certain amount of rest in order for our bodies to recharge and recover. When that's missing, our body moves towards dis-ease. We also need specific nutrients and minerals.

When we lack them... well... our bodies don't work like they're designed. And, remember, **we can "eat right" and still miss some of the much needed nutrients.** Again, good food isn't enough.

CAUSES OF DIS-EASE

	EXPLAINED	EXAMPLES
TOXINS	Too much of something that should not be present	Stress, sugar, scented candles, etc.
DEFICIENCIES	Too little of something that should be present	Sleep, nutrients

---

[159] Remember, this is why your body seeks to eliminate glucose (sugar) from your system as quickly as possible.

Start with your gut

So, the question looms, How do we fix this? If food is not enough for optimal health, what do we do?

Here's the answer: *start with your gut.*

The gut is often referred to as the "second brain." The gut has as many neurons as the brain of a small pet, so if a dog is intelligent... well... so is your stomach.[160]

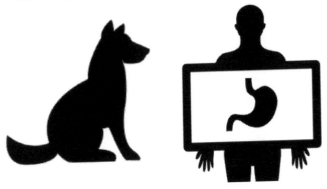

Turns out, gut health is one of the greatest factors determining your overhaul health and wellbeing. The saying "You are what you eat" is true.

Here are a few of the most important functions of the gut:

---

[160] See the film, *The Gut: Our Second Brain,* available on Amazon Prime.

- Your immune system (80% of it!) is largely housed in the gut.[161]

- Your cardiovascular health and many of your major organs are tied to the gut.

- Your gut's condition determines what your body can do with the nutrients you take in- including the nutrients you ingest from food and from supplements.

While researching this information, I spoke to a staff member at Young Living, the brand of supplements and nutritional products we recommend. She said, "People have to care for their gut and get it healthy first. If you eat right and take supplements but your gut is in such poor shape that it can't digest them, well... it won't make that much of a difference."

Let me be graphically blunt: you can invest a lot of money in incredible supplements. But if your body can't access them because your stomach isn't able to digest the nutrients, you'll just "poop them out."

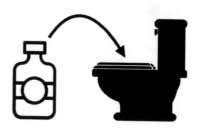

This creates a dilemma.

On one hand, "once you fix your digestive issues, you will experience a surge of energy, weight loss, and clarity of mind, enthusiasm, and clear

---

[161] Dr. LeAnne Deardeuff and Dr. David Deardeuff, *Inner Transformations Using Essential Oils*, p175.

skin. Depression and anxiety will begin to go away."[162] That is, fuel your body in the right way and many of the health issues we've learned to tolerate will vanish.

On the other hand, though, good food *still* is not enough. We need support from products like MultiGreens. But, if our body can't leverage the nutrition from those precious resources, we're not going to be much that much better off.

Enter Life 9.

Life 9

Life 9 is a probiotic. *Pro* **means it's "for" the "biotics," that is, living organisms. You recognize the opposite of this word:** *antibiotics.* **Antibiotics kill bacteria. The problem with antibiotics is that they indiscriminately kill** *all* **bacteria in your body. Your health, however, actually depends on the presence of good bacteria-** *particularly in your digestive system.*

Your digestive tract is 30-feet long. Each segment features a different method of breaking down specific forms of food into fuel for your body.[163]

---

162 Dr. LeAnne Deardeuff and Dr. David Deardeuff, *Inner Transformations Using Essential Oils*, p175.

163 Source: https://www.asge.org/home/about-asge/newsroom/media-backgrounders-detail/human-digestive-system, accessed 10-07-2017.

Life 9 features 17 billion live cultures from 9 beneficial strands of bacteria (hence, the name). The beauty of Life 9, though, is that its created with "delayed-time release" functionality. That means it deploys the live cultures throughout your intestine at the specific places in your intestine where the different strands are needed the most. This is important, because if they're released too early or too late at any point along that 30-foot journey, they could die, making them of no value to your body.

Sounds high tech, doesn't it?

Some people suggest you should eat yogurt- that it contains some degree of probiotics. However, read the label. Most "yogurt" is just milk and sugar. Furthermore, sugar actually suppresses your immune system! And, sugar causes your body to release insulin, thereby promoting fat storage in your body.

So far I've recommended two supplements to you. Neither one is free. This leads to one of the most common misconceptions about good health...

The cost issue

A lot of people decide that health products- like supplements- are too expensive. In fact, a lot of people believe the misconception that better food is more expensive, too. If you look just at the "sticker price" *only* you might believe this myth, too.

Let's dig deeper...

It's not uncommon to see obese people who are actually malnourished.[164] This is because of the following:

- Bad food often *appears* cheaper than good food.

- Bad food has a sticker price that's *definitely lower* than the price of good food.

- Bad food contains calories but has no nutritional value.

- Your body can't absorb non-nutrients, yet it *craves* nutrition. When you eat food with no nutritional value, your body doesn't feel as if it's eaten. You aren't satisfied, so you crave more (and you continue eating).

The dilemma is that *all calories* add weight to your body- whether they're healthy calories or unhealthy ones. Yet calories are "not all created equal." Whereas calories from living foods are easy for your body to breakdown into nutritional fuel (you eat and find yourself satisfied), calories from processed foods aren't easily broken down. They tend to pack weight on, even as they leave you unsatisfied and hungry for more.[165]

I've heard several health practitioners say something like this: **You can pay "a little more" now to enjoy health, or you can pay "a lot more" later to fix your un-health.**

We've learned this firsthand:

- In the short term, you'll actually spend *about the same amount* of money on healthy food as unhealthy food. You'll

---

[164] See the documentary *Fat, Sick, and Nearly Dead* (http://www.fatsickandnearlydead.com).

[165] In chapter 8 of the book we discuss hunger hormones- and how carbs (read: glucose / sugar) throw them out of whack, making you crave more junk food.

need far less of the better food. It's nutrient-dense and actually works *with* your body.

- In the long term, you'll spend *far less* on health, because you'll avoid the costly issues associated with obesity and other forms of dis-ease. [166]

Good food and good health is actually financially cheaper than bad health. Aside from the savings, good health actually "feels better," too.

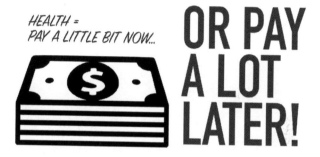

HEALTH =
PAY A LITTLE BIT NOW... **OR PAY A LOT LATER!**

Helpful Hints for Advanced Users

In addition to Life 9...

---

[166] I struggled with referring to obesity as a dis-ease. Remember our definition, though: dis-ease is caused by deficiencies ("not enough" of good things your body needs) or toxins (too much of something that it doesn't). Excess weight is something your body does not need; it's a toxin. In fact, the AMA has publicly recognized obesity as a disease. See the following: http://www.nytimes.com/2013/06/19/business/ama-recognizes-obesity-as-a-disease.html , http://newsroom.heart.org/news/american-medical-association-says-obesity-is-a-disease , http://www.npr.org/sections/health-shots/2013/06/19/193440570/ama-says-its-time-to-call-obesity-a-disease

- If you have food intolerances, add Alerzyme to your daily routine. This product is great for people who are lactose intolerant, gluten intolerant, or suffer from Irritable Bowel Syndrome and bloating.

- If you have trouble absorbing nutrients, add Ezzentialzyme-4 to your routine. This product is a prebiotic, designed to be ingested before you eat. In turn, it drives the nutrients deep into your body systems, helping you absorb them.

- If you suffer from allergies (and even "hangovers" from certain food ands and drinks), try Detoxzyme as part of your routine.

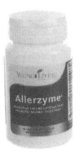 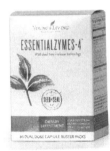 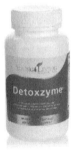

Hidden health issues

Again, the first imperative is to solve problems associated with your gut (using a probiotic like Life 9). Remember, you've got to get your body in a place where it can absorb the nutrients it desperately needs. Then, once your body can absorb the nutrients it needs, you need to flood your body with those nutrients (i.e., MultiGreens). These steps alone, coupled with eating right, will solve many of your health concerns.

However, we're all unique. Sometimes, "hidden" problems persist. By that, I mean something happens that we can't really explain. The issues are so familiar that we come to expect them. **The solution to many of these nuisances that we learn to "tolerate" is often remedied by supporting the thyroid.**

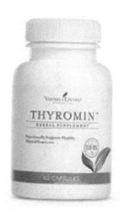

For instance, many people complain that they have a hard time losing or gaining weight.[167] (That second group is a bit annoying, aren't they? "I can eat anything I want and don't gain a thing!")

This *might* be a thyroid issue.[168] You see:

- An over-active thyroid prevents you from being able to gain weight

- An under-active thyroid prevents you from being able to lose weight

In other words, **the thyroid effects your digestive system because it alters your metabolism.** Food is fuel. Your digestive system is tied to your ability to do something with that fuel, to run all the processes necessary to keep your body alive.[169] So, if you've got "hidden" and

---

[167] First, make sure you are eating right. Read through the Keto book and make sure you're eating the correct macros.

[168] For more info, go to https://en.wikipedia.org/wiki/Hyperthyroidism

[169] Metabolism isn't just "the rate of how fast or slow you burn food." Metabolism includes all of your "life processes," including breathing, circulation, muscular regeneration, etc.

"unexplained" health concerns, this is the second place to look (after starting with your gut).

Let's put it in terms we can all relate to- outside of our bodies: Think about how functional your car would be if too much gas ran through the engine too quickly (over-active) OR if the fuel was diverted somewhere besides the engine. Your car might run, but it certainly wouldn't run and peak performance levels.

Other people struggle with chronic fatigue. They find themselves consistently tired- or more tired than they feel they should be in light of their work load. An under-active thyroid can cause this. Too much fuel stays in the tank rather than running through the engine and converting to energy. You feel like you're "out of gas" when, oddly enough, the tank remains completely full.

(Remember, an under-active thyroid also makes it difficult to lose weight. So, it's possible to find yourself feeling stuck in a cycle of being "fat and tired.")

Finally, many people can't get their core body temperature quite right. If your thyroid is under-active, you'll find yourself hot. Add this to the other issues of an under-active thyroid (feeling obese and tired) and you've got the trifecta. [170]

Notice the chart below. The first line (Over-active) describes some people. They're unusually skinny. They have specific bursts of energy, but regularly crash. They feel chilly- even when it's warm.

The second line, though, describes a lot of people. Overweight- and can't seem to shake it. Consistently tired. Always hot and miserable. If you relate, perhaps the thyroid is an issue you need to address.

---

[170] Side note: one YL exec told me that many times women who experience "hot flashes" may actually be dealing with thyroid issues. Her point was this: an unhealthy thyroid can also mess with your menstrual cycles.

PROBLEMS ASSOCIATED WITH THYROID HEALTH

	WEIGHT	FATIGUE	BODY TEMP
OVER-ACTIVE	Can't gain weight	Bursts of energy, then crash	Always feel cold
UNDER-ACTIVE	Can't lose weight	Consistently tired	Always feel hot

No one likes to spend $30 for an oil change every 3,000 miles- or 3 months. Over the course of a year, that's $120 that could go towards some other (seemingly more important) budget item, right?

But a new engine costs well over $3,000. And that's exactly what cars that don't receive oil changes eventually require- a complete overhaul!

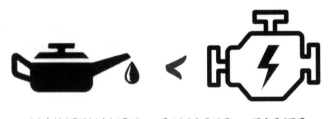

MAINTENANCE = CHEAPER + EASIER

In the same way, **yes, health costs a little bit. But, un-health costs far more**. Dis-ease is a price that I'm no longer willing to pay.

That leads us to our second core idea...

Core idea 2: Your body is self-healing

Your body's natural state is actually health. You may not feel healthy right now, but- I promise- your body's natural state is health. Remember, the foundational causes of all dis-ease have to do with toxins (things that shouldn't be present) or deficiencies (things that need to be present).

Consider...

- Your body has an immune system- 80% of which is housed in your gut. Your body does *not* have a disease system that manufactures illness.

- Your blood stream houses T-white blood cells, courageous fighters that literally war against dis-ease on your behalf. In fact, when infection enters, they "call in" reinforcements and multiply in number.

- Your bones will mend if broken (often healing more rigid than they were before the break), your skin will repair itself when cut, and your colon will expel food you eat that upsets the balance of your digestive system.

When you provide your body with the best possible environment you can (one that is lower in toxins and has the nutrients in needs), your body becomes extremely efficient at optimizing health. This is because when you create this environment in your body, you actually create space where your body can do what it wants to do automatically.

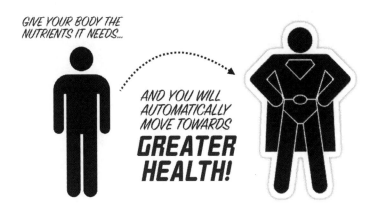

That leads us to another product your body needs to create this environment of wellness…

OmegaGize

Let me introduce you to one of my favorite supplements, OmegaGize.

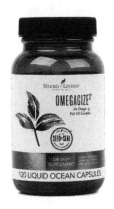

One of the key ingredients of OmegaGize is Omega-3 fatty acid / fish oil, the same fatty acid in our brains. In fact, there's widespread agreement about this: "It's the one thing we doctors who embrace natural strategies for health have in agreement with mainstream cardiologists."[171]

---

[171] See Suzanne Somers, *Breakthrough*, p328.

Fish oil is essential for brain health *and* cardiac health. It improves your blood flow, as it helps your blood maintain the consistency of wine rather than ketchup. (Sugar actually thickens blood. Thick, sticky blood isn't healthy.)[172]

As well, OmegaGize also features CoQ10, a co-enzyme. Co-enxymes work with your body's natural enzymes in order to help them perform more efficiently. One of the most important is Coenzyme Q10. This co-enzyme is found in *every cell* of the body.[173] CoQ10 is actually made naturally by the body in order to support normal cellular function and energy production- particularly for the heart, liver, and kidneys. But, CoQ10 levels naturally decline with age.

CoQ10 is also naturally present in small amounts in a wide variety of foods- particularly foods considered to be higher in fat (like meats and nuts).[174] Remember what we learned in the beginning of this chapter, though- even good food isn't enough.

Why is all of this important? Well you *need* fat in your body. And the co-enzymes that accompany it.

The "low fat" movement boomed in the early 1980s because everyone thought *fat* was bad. As a result, they eliminated fat from almost all foods.[175] Turns out, not only does your body *need* fat, but fat also makes food taste good. In order to remedy the problem of "tasteless" food, manufacturers began adding high doses of sugar into everything. In other words, **they removed something your body needs (creating**

---

[172] Suzanne Somers, *Breakthrough*, p327.

[173] https://www.webmd.com/heart-disease/heart-failure/tc/coenzyme-q10-topic-overview#1

[174] https://www.webmd.com/heart-disease/heart-failure/tc/coenzyme-q10-topic-overview#1

[175] It turns out that the sugar industry engineered the studies throughout that era in order to label fat as the culprit. See http://www.businessinsider.com/sugar-health-effects-body-brain-2016-9. See chapter 3 of this book for more on the history of Keto.

a deficiency), and they added something your body doesn't need (creating a toxin!).

The excessive use of refined sugar (the toxin of all toxins!) unleashed a litany of problems, including things like:

- Risks of high blood pressure

- Insatiable hunger (You aren't satisfied, since sugar provides you with "empty calories" and hijacks your hunger cravings, so your body desires even more, leading you to binge more.)

- Kidney disease (Ever wondered why there are so many dialysis clinics popping up in shopping centers lately? Yeah, all the sugar we're eating has a lot to do with it!)

- Weight gain (One study suggests that the average male adult will lose 20-25 pounds per year simply by eliminating sugar from his drinks- even if he changes *nothing else* about his diet or exercise patterns.)[176]

Many of the substitutes we use to replace sugar (aspartame, stevia, etc.) have even *more* and *greater* side effects than sugar! In other words, by making fat the culprit we've opened ourselves to sugar... then by seeing the ills of sugar we've (many times) moved to even worse products!

Again, *your body needs fat*. It actually craves it. It's good for you!

How good is it? Well...

---

[176] This goes back to the idea I mentioned earlier, that diet may actually be more important than exercise- assuming you had to choose between one or the other. Thankfully, we don't. We can utilize both in our quest for optimal health.

Your brain actually requires fat to function, as do your lungs. Your brain is 60% fat, as our the linings of your neurological cells.

As well, in a sense, fat "greases" your system and keep the parts moving. (Ever heard of a collapsed lung? Many times that happens because the lungs stick together- there's no lubrication.)

Yes, fat looks nasty in a jar- just like the grease in your car's engine. But, without these ingredients, you (and your car) don't function...

So what do the fatty acids in OmegaGize do?

They "grease" the digestive process. They lubricate the skeletal muscles. They support your digestive processes, your heart, your eyes, your skin, and your joints. In other words, they help keep the "engine" operational.

Now, let me introduce you to the fourth supplement on my "must have" list...

NingXia Red

NingXia Red is a drink derived from the wolfberry. It's name honors the NingXia province of Northern China, the one place on earth where the small red berry is grown and harvested.

Wolfberries are known as *phyto-nutrients- phyto* coming from the Greek word for "plant" and *nutrient* denoting the fuel your body needs for optimal health.

What are *phyto-nutrients*? Quite simply, they're their own category of superfoods. They're not carbs, proteins, or fats... they're plant based fuel. This fuel contains an ample supply of many of the nutrients your body needs in a highly dense package.

Let me walk you through a few of the key components of NingXia Red, as that will help illustrate how the Red works. I'll tell you about potassium, zinc, and amino acids.

First, NingXia Red is loaded with potassium, one of the key components necessary for the function of all living cells. Potassium is responsible for:

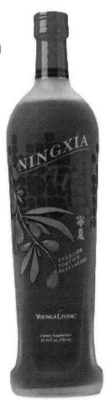

- Hormone secretion

- Heart tone and blood pressure control

- Glucose and insulin metabolism

- Renal / kidney ability

- Fluid and electrolyte balance

- Cognitive health

In other words, *potassium is essential to life.*

The problem, though, is that *your body doesn't manufacture it* (as it does with CoQ10). You have to "get it" somewhere.[177] Turns out, the wolf berry, the key ingredient in NingXia Red, is one of the highest sources of potassium known to man.

Second, NingXia Red is full of zinc- one of the major factors in overall immune support for your body. If I offered my kids a handful of Brussel sprouts each morning, they'd refuse. If I

---

[177] The actual term for this is "essential," meaning it's essential that you ingest it if you're going to have it.

asked them to drink a raw egg (like Rocky Balboa), they'd pitch a fit. Now, get this comparison: NingXia Red boosts 5x the amount of zinc found in a serving of Brussel sprouts, as well as 5x the mount of zinc found in a raw egg- all in a single 1 ounce serving.

(That's right. Catch that "1 ounce" part. You don't drink NingXia by the glass. You only need "a shot" of the Red to get the benefits. It's that nutritionally dense.)

Third, wolfberries contain every essential amino acid your body needs for optimal function. With 13 percent protein content, wolfberries offer one of the highest protein levels of any fruit. This, too, is vital for cellular health and immune support. And it demonstrates that you don't have to eat a stack of meat in order to reach your protein quota for the day.

I use Red as a pre-workout energy boost, to supply the "on demand" energy my muscles need when called into action. We give it to our kids as a pre-day dose of immune support. *This is part of our daily routine.*

Quick review

In closing, let's review two of the core ideas of this chapter.

First, the root causes of all dis-ease is one of the following: toxins and deficiencies. By now, you remember that a toxin is something that should not be in your body but is, and a deficiency is something you need that isn't present in great enough quantity.

Notice that there's an inverse relationship between toxicity and nutrition:

- Higher levels of toxins = Greater level of deficiencies (read: minimal nutrition) = LOWER overall health

- Lower levels of toxins = Lower level of deficiencies (read: nutrition) = GREATER overall health

Toxicity vs. Nutrients

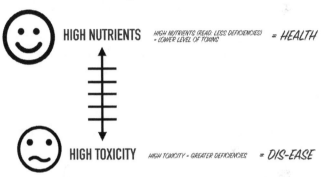

Notice that when we're walking in unhealthy patterns "the nutrient levels go down and the toxicity levels go up."[178] On the other hand, **when we're experiencing health, it's because the nutrients have gone up and the toxins have gone down.** We continue moving higher above the wellness line when we create an environment of nutrition.

(By the way, the more toxins you have in your body, the more fat your body needs to store them. This is why you can binge sugar for the weekend and instantly feel like you have an extra layer of fat on your love handles or your thighs. More toxins present = more storage containers needed to handle the extra load.[179])

---

[178] Suzanne Somers, *Tox-Sick*, p127.

[179] Suzanne Sommers, *Tox-Sick*, p154.

Second, your body is self-healing. If you create an environment based on the above (eliminating toxins and shoring-up the deficiencies), you'll naturally move towards increased health.

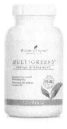 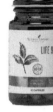 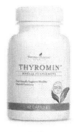 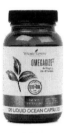 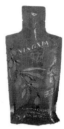

| *FOOD IS NOT ENOUGH* | *DIGESTIVE, IMMUNE SUPPORT, NUTRIENT DELIVERY* | *HIDDEN HEALTH ISSUES* | *HEART + COGNITIVE + CELLULAR* | *REBUILD + REPLENISH* |

The core four supplements I recommend to create this environment of health are-

- MultiGreens

- Life 9 (probiotic)

- OmegaGize (fish oil supplement)

- NingXia Red (overall fitness)

Of course, in addition to these, you may also be a prime candidate for Thyromin (thyroid health).

How to get your own products

Yes, there is a cost to living well- but *everything* has a cost. The cost of not doing something is *greater*.

Remember the oil change vs. new engine cost comparison? Yeah, there's not really a financial comparison at all when you compare the true numbers, right?

And, of course, choosing not to do something is in actuality a decision- it's a choice to continue living with toxins and deficiencies, all while *the opportunity to walk in greater health is available.*

Imagine what life will be like when you wake up ready to face your day! When you aren't sluggish in the afternoon! When the foods you eat provide fuel and energy to your body, rather than excessive bloating, gas, and stomach issues…

You're at a crossroads and can choose one path or the other.

We recommend Young Living essential oils and products. In fact, **Young Living is the *only* company where you can purchase the products I've recommended. They're *exclusive* to this one company.** Continue reading, and I'll tell you how to get the best price, so that you can begin living your best life now.

You're in one of two camps at this point-

- You either already have Young Living essential oils- and are a wholesale member, *OR*

- You're not one yet

(By the way, wholesale membership doesn't tie you down to buying something every week, every month, or even every year for the rest of your life. Nor does it sign you up for auto-ship or any other kind of contract. It simply means you get THE BEST prices on THE BEST products. AND, unlike Sam's or Costco where you pay a fee to become a member and have the right to shop but don't get any actual products, the way to become a wholesale member of Young Living is to actually make a wholesale purchase!)

Let's go back to the two groups of people I just mentioned...

First, let's discuss the first group, current members. If you currently have a wholesale membership with Young Living, the best option for you is to purchase the products directly through your wholesale member account. Since you're already a member, you can get this for the best price, at wholesale (24% off retail).[180]

Second, let's discuss the second group, those who aren't members yet. The best option for you is to become a member, so that you don't pay $60-plus MORE than wholesale members.

You can become a member in TWO ways.

- **Option 1 to become a member: Purchase a "basic membership" ($45.00) and add the products to your order.** This brings your total cost to $285 (including Thyromin) or $243.25 (without Thyromin)- *far less than you'd pay for retail.*[181] Plus, you can purchase at any time in the future with wholesale pricing! Oh, and you receive the following:

  - One bottle of Stress Away essential oil (the name says it all)

  - Two additional on-the-go servings of NingXia Red

- **Option 2 to become a member: Purchase the Premium Starter Kit (pictured on the following page).** The PSK includes the 11 of the most popular oils, a diffuser, and 2 servings of NingXia Red. The total retail value is OVER $330, making this an amazing deal at $170. If you're doing

---

[180] Just login to your virtual office. I've listed the products and item numbers below.

[181] Note: these prices are current as of the publish date of this book. Prices are subject to change.

the math, you'll notice that this is just $135 more than the basic kit-

By the way, each of these products comes from Young Living as a monthly supply- a plus when you're budgeting and trying to figure out if you'll have enough supplements to make it through the week, right?

Premium Starter Kit

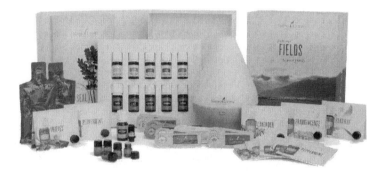

Why become a wholesale member?

Either way you choose (the basic membership or the Premium Starter Kit with the 12 essential oils + diffuser),

- **You get the best products on the planet.**

- **You become part of an amazing community, full of people who are learning to walk in health +**

wholeness. Though we come from a variety of backgrounds, we have this journey in common. And, we support one another and encourage each other through our private Facebook groups.

- **You'll have access to some of the best resources anywhere.** With our regular Zoom calls, webinars, and online classes, you'll have great info to continue learning life-changing truths just like you're learning now. All of these are *free* to our team members.

- **Here's one of the best parts: wholesale members receive a 24% discount on ALL of their purchases AND they're eligible for free products every single month**.

- **This final one is THE MOST IMPORTANT ONE, though:** *You.* The best version of you is just on the other side of accessing these great resources.

For ordering info call / text 205-291-1391

MEMBERSHIP + SUPPLEMENT OPTIONS

	Item #	Retail $	Basic Core Four	Basic + One More	Premium Core Four	Premium + One More
MEMBERSHIP			$45.00	$45.00	$160.00	$160.00
MULTIGREENS	#3248 (120ct)	$52.30	$39.75	$39.75	$39.75	$39.75
LIFE 9	#18299 (30ct)	$37.83	$28.75	$28.75	$28.75	$28.75
OMEGAGIZE	#3097 (120ct)	$77.30	$58.75	$58.75	$58.75	$58.75
NINGXIA RED	#3042 (2x 750 ml)	$93.42	$71.00	$71.00	$71.00	$71.00
THYROMIN	#3246 (60ct)	$54.93		$41.75		$41.75
TOTAL		$315.78	$243.25	$285.00	$358.25	$400.00

D. OTHER RESOURCES

Books

Keto Clarity, Jimmy Moore

The Ketogenic Diet, Kristen Mancinelli

Dr. Colbert's Keto Zone Diet, Don Colbert

The Bulletproof Diet, Dave Asprey

Eat Fat, Get Thin, Mark Hyman

What You Need to Know About Keto, Tom Nikkola

Wheat Belly, William Davis

Films / documentaries

Cereal Killers: Don't Eat Fat (www.CerealKillersMovie.com)

Fat Head (Tom Naughton, www.Fathhead-movie.com)

Fat, Sick, & Nearly Dead (Joe Cross, Kurt Ergfehr, FatSickAndNearlyDead.com)

Run on Fat: Cereal Killers 2 (www.RunOnFatMovie.com)

That Sugar Film (www.ThatSugarFilm.com)

Podcasts*

2 Keto Dudes

Ben Greenfield Fitness

Fit 2 Fat 2 Fit Experience

The Ketovangelist Podcast

Note: most of these podcasts have accompanying websites

Websites

FindingKeto.online

DietDoctor.com

Ketogasm.com (Keto for women)

LivanLaVidaLowCarb.com

Ruled.me

Access the audiobook + bonus content at www.FindingKeto.online

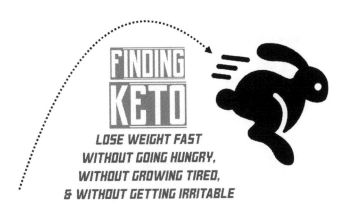

FINDING KETO

LOSE WEIGHT FAST WITHOUT GOING HUNGRY, WITHOUT GROWING TIRED, & WITHOUT GETTING IRRITABLE

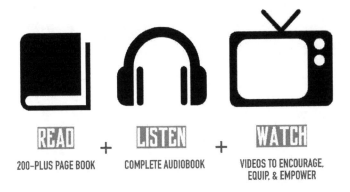

READ + **LISTEN** + **WATCH**

200-PLUS PAGE BOOK   COMPLETE AUDIOBOOK   VIDEOS TO ENCOURAGE, EQUIP, & EMPOWER

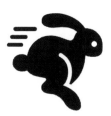

Unless you've been living like a hermit for the past few years, you've probably heard of Keto- a "new" diet craze that's en vogue.

But Keto isn't new. In fact, the low-carb-high-fat plan of nutrition was actually prescribed by doctors in the U.S. to treat epilepsy and neurological disorders less than a century ago. And it was used throughout Europe to heal degenerative body diseases.

So why has it resurged in popularity? And is it right for you?

In Finding Keto, we talk- from firsthand experience- about the nutrition plan that empowers you to lose weight AND works FOR your health. Let's face it: a lot of weight loss programs don't. In some sense, many diet plans for you to choose between losing weight or being healthy. Or between losing weight and starving. Or between losing weight and having more energy.

Keto works with your body's need for fats, enabling you to melt the fat off your body all while having more energy, thinking more clearly, and enriching your mood.

Keto works WITH your body's natural nutrient needs and facilitates rapid weight loss- all while allowing you to NOT go hungry, NOT grow tired, and NOT get irritable.

Backed by science and real world experience, Finding Keto outlines practical steps you can take to evaluate if the ketogenic diet is for you, as well as begin the Keto lifestyle immediately.

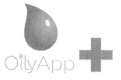